# STEPPING INTO MORE

Lessons from a Recovering Perfectionist

*Rachel Karu, MS, ACC*

STEPPING INTO MORE

Copyright © 2012 by Rachel Karu, MS, ACC

All rights reserved. No part of this book may be reproduced or transmitted in any form or by any means without written permission of the author.

ISBN 9781624076374

# Acknowledgments

To my loving husband Ron for his unwavering support and his graciousness in agreeing to share our story. He is the sweetest soul I have ever met.

To my children – truly the biggest blessings in my life. Thanks for accepting me for me and allowing me to be the best mom I know how to be by providing me with space and understanding as I take time to nurture myself and pursue my creative endeavors.

To my parents – for bringing me into this world and for teaching me so many life lessons.

# Contents

| | | |
|---|---|---|
| Prologue | | 1 |
| 1. | My American Pie | 5 |
| 2. | A Star is Born | 12 |
| 3. | From Method Acting to Singing Telegram | 23 |
| 4. | Two Weddings and a Business Degree | 31 |
| 5. | I Dreamed a Dream | 43 |
| 6. | This Land is Your Land, This Land is My Land?? | 54 |
| 7. | I'm an Adult Now | 63 |
| 8. | Take Me Out to the Ball Game | 72 |
| 9. | I Did It My Way! | 85 |
| 10. | I Am Woman | 96 |
| 11. | The Accident That Was No Accident | 103 |
| 12. | Please Don't Stop the Music | 110 |
| 13. | Defying Gravity | 120 |
| 14. | Breaking Through | 129 |
| 15. | No More Wheaties for Me! | 143 |
| 16. | This is Me in All My Glory | 148 |
| 17. | You Know You Make Me Want to Shout! | 157 |
| 18. | Reality Song: What are the Lessons and Can I Learn Them Already?! | 169 |
| 19. | Living My Dream All Along | 179 |
| 20. | A New Chapter Begins – the Best is Yet to Come | 190 |

# Prologue

I was 17 years old on a summer day, sitting in my apartment in Van Nuys California that I shared with my friend Eydie. It was an ordinary afternoon. I recently started summer break after spending a year studying at the American Academy of Dramatic Arts. I was the youngest student at the time. Happy to be on vacation, I was enjoying the lazy afternoon when I decided to take a walk to the mail box. I came upstairs and settled into the couch prepared to peruse the junk mail and the latest bills.

As I fumbled through the mail, I noticed a letter from the American Academy of Dramatic Arts. My heart started pounding heavily as I realized this letter would seal my fate for the next year and possibly forever. I was eagerly waiting to find out if I was accepted into the second year program. The last year was a rollercoaster ride of emotions as I delved into various classes – method acting, singing, diction, dance, just to name a few. I experienced great highs as well as many moments of self-doubt and fear. I was pretty certain I would go back – I just had an inner knowing. I paused and took a deep breath before I ripped open the letter.

To my shock and horror, I learned that I had been rejected to the second year program. It was the standard form letter, not much explanation. I felt the tears well up and a wave of shame running through my body. I suddenly felt nauseous and I had a million, thoughts running through my head.

> "How could this have happened?"
> "You are a pathetic loser."
> "I can't fathom telling anyone about this disgraceful news."
> "What the hell am I going to do with my life?"

In my Perfectionist mind, my fate was decided. I would never be a performer. I obviously lacked the talent and I was completely embarrassed. I quickly determined that my future was ruined and all my dreams had ended at the tender age of 17.

After a few months working for my Dad in his check cashing stores (I could write a whole book about this experience), I regrouped and decided to take the path more frequently travelled by attending college and studying business. I would please my family and lead a "normal" respectable life.

After college I embarked on my career as a Human Resources and personal and professional development manager and specialist. I compartmentalized my life into four major categories: 1) Business professional 2) Creative person 3) Family member, 4) Friend. I felt a bit schizophrenic, experiencing multiple personalities as I behaved quite differently in each role. One theme was consistent with each role – my Perfectionist was in the driver's seat. She created many rules and I made most choices based on the fear she instilled in me.

My dream to perform did indeed die for over 23 years until about six years ago when my life took an unexpected turn. I experienced an unusual series of events which I will share with you during this memoir and guide. This journey forced me to re-assess my life and led me to *Stepping into More* by shifting from being a Perfectionist to a Recovering Perfectionist.

You are about to read my voyage and learn how I:

- consciously chose a path of integration versus compartmentalization
- learned to feel the fear and do it anyway
- discovered how to come full circle with my performing and share my voice in a meaningful way
- pulled off my masks and let my gentle strength be my guiding light

## How the Book is Written

I have been a personal and professional development coach, trainer, consultant, and speaker as well as an undiscovered singer for more than 18 years. In my usual Recovering Perfectionist way, I tried to approach writing this book as I do most things – with much structure and form. I decided I would write an outline and have it all figured out before I started writing; that would provide me with the illusion of control that I could have the whole book wrapped up in a neat package with a clear ending – before the journey had even begun.

It didn't take me long to realize that this book would flow through me, I could not control the story, and I had no idea if there would be a happy ending when I completed it. I was determined and committed to completing this project so most of the writing took place during 15-20 minute chunks at 5:15 a.m. when I woke before the rest of my household and could get some focused time. This has been a labor of love.

I am passionate about inspiring reflection and results in myself and others. I hope that you can find yourself in this story and reclaim your values, passions, and dreams. My wish is that my story and its lessons will assist you on your own journey and give you the strength to stand authentically in your power (flaws and all), and bring all of who you are to your life and work.

I ended each chapter with a section titled **Lessons Learned** to help draw out the universal messages that can support you. I also included a section **Deepen Your Learning** where I provide questions and inquiries for you to answer to support you in applying the concepts and tools I share. I hope that my story touches and inspires you to reflect and take meaningful action. I wish you a good read!

# 1
## My American Pie

"I was born a poor black child." I always loved that line from the movie, "The Jerk," but alas, that isn't part of my story. What is more accurate is the observation made by my Great Aunt Rose (may she rest in peace) who reminded me that I had sung before I could speak. At the age of five, I was belting out Don McLean's "American Pie" and Sonny and Cher's "Cherokee People." In other words, I was born to sing.

Singing always created a safe outlet for me to emote – especially strong emotions like sadness, loneliness or anger. Like most kids, I had my share of those feelings, but our family moved a lot and that made matters much worse. Whenever my dad had a good business opportunity, we moved. Those moves definitely impacted my feelings of security, or should I say insecurity.

I was born in Brooklyn, New York and moved to Lawrence Park, NY at the tender age of one. Not long after that, we moved to a house in Rockland County, NY and then to Florida when I was five. We hit Oklahoma when I was eight and Los Angeles, California just before my twelfth birthday.

Singing and music helped me get through some of those tough times; it was soothing and cathartic. In kindergarten, I stood holding on to the monkey bars by myself at recess, singing and crying. I don't even remember what I was singing or why I was crying. I held onto the cold metal bars, feeling so alone in the world, my body rhythmically moving to the song. I discovered that I could use singing to soothe myself.

When I was about nine years old, our school had a talent contest. I came up with the idea of singing a song even though I had never performed before (unless you count a group rendition of "Kumbaya" in my kindergarten talent show!) I chose "When I Need You" by Leo Sayer as a tribute to — and an expression of love for — my dad, who traveled a great deal. He was really my hero at that point in my life; I had him seated high up on a pedestal. My mom always had a difficult time expressing her love for me. She was strict, set many rules, and was very emotional. I don't blame her – her parents were very difficult people. I can now see that it must have been extremely hard for her to act as a single parent while my dad was on the road.

But I didn't see things so clearly when I was a little girl. In contrast to my mom, my dad openly showed affection toward me – not only would he say nice things, he would also hug and tickle me. Of course, I worshiped him since his approach was in such stark contrast to my mother's.

I practiced the song regularly with the record player (that was before the CD era) in our living room with the shag carpet (that my dad used to rake!). I felt the sadness of missing my dad and wished he could be at home more often. But performing that song *a cappella* in the little chapel at our synagogue left me feeling wonderful about the whole experience (even if my dad wasn't in the audience).

I later auditioned for a solo song in a school play but didn't get the part. Feeling embarrassed and ashamed, I didn't want to participate at all. In spite of my feelings, I did end up accepting a lesser role and sticking with the play. Now, in retrospect, I can see that my Perfectionism was rearing its head. If I didn't get the lead (or the part I desired), then I felt I "shouldn't" participate at all; it was all or nothing.

I developed the need to be both seen and heard at a very early age. While our perpetual relocating forced me to create new friends often, I also felt somewhat invisible within my own family. My younger brother Adam and I were subject to the whims of my dad's moves and my mother's rules and moods. I wasn't given much of a voice in our house; I was supposed to do what my parents told me without questioning or complaining. There was an unspoken rule that the children were expected to follow the rules and appear to be happy. My parents didn't like it when I was overtly angry, inquisitive or sad…except for when I sang! That was the only time they were okay with my expressing any less-than-positive emotions.

I learned early on that my voice moved people and that generated a sense of inner power. Singing became my "secret weapon." We could be in a crowded room or an airport and I knew that if I chose to sing, the room would go silent and I would be heard.

In fact, self-expression and the need to be heard continue to be key values for me. As an adult, I still struggle with the difference between "having a voice" and feeling obligated to lead, to be in charge. I am still reconciling my urge to be heard with the knowledge that I don't always have to be responsible for making things happen.

The title of this memoir and guide – *Stepping into More*, is all about the process of grappling with our various aspects and learning how to make clear choices. Throughout the story you will hear me refer to three aspects of myself "The Three Ps": the Perfectionist Gremlin, the Performer, and the Professional:

My Perfectionist Gremlin experiences life as…
- *black and white*
- *wrong and right*
- *bleak and sad*
- *scary and overwhelming*
- *scarce and cruel*
- *needing to protect me by playing small*
- *placing high expectations on myself and others*
- *beating myself up*
- *perpetual negative tapes running in my head*
- *angry*

- *lonely and gray*
- *win or lose*
- *needing approval and validation from the outside*
- *a shitty day*

My Performer experiences life as...
- *recognizing each moment is a gift*
- *knowing how to enjoy what is*
- *being connected to the situation and the people with me*
- *following my intuition and instincts*
- *trusting that I know exactly what I need to do in any given moment*
- *leading from my heart instead of my head*
- *being vulnerable*
- *sharing my gentle strength*
- *knowing each day is a fresh start*
- *loving and accepting myself as I am*
- *accepting others without high expectations*
- *being flexible and adaptable*

My Professional experiences life as...
- *wearing a mask*
- *living a persona*
- *being polite and diplomatic – sometimes to a fault*
- *holding back my truth*
- *sacrificing myself to meet others' needs*
- *trying to fit into someone else's image of who I should be*
- *knowing what to say and do in order to "fit in" with any given situation*

I can alternate between these different profiles during a single conversation, and can feel all "three P's" coming into play when I perform. While preparing for a performance, I experience a conflict between the Performer and the Perfectionist Gremlin (from this point forward I will refer to this aspect of myself as Perfectionist. I will discuss the concept of Gremlins in more detail below): My Performer wants to create music from the heart and to trust my instincts about remembering the lyrics and connecting with the audience. My Perfectionist imagines an empty house, worries about presenting a package that will please everyone, is sure I won't remember the lyrics and doubts my talent.

Just before going onstage, I can feel myself struggling with the fear that I won't be able to let go and hear my Performer voice, the one that will serve me best throughout the show.

As an adult on stage, I tend to vacillate between all three. I am certainly the Professional as I am speaking to the audience and sharing my "patter" in between songs. I am energetic, polite and polished. I script out what I will say and pretty much stick to what I have planned. I know when my Performer has shown up because that's when I will improvise or suddenly make a funny remark. I am in tuned with what is going on in the moment and I follow my intuition and speak freely. My Performer is also at play when I acknowledge and make light of any mistakes that have occurred during the show. I am in my ultimate Performer zone when I am singing and allowing myself to feel the music. I am breathing deeply and feeling a warm sensation over my heart and in my hands; my body is moving freely and I am at ease. Those are the moments I cherish.

And then suddenly, in the middle of a song, my Perfectionist rears up and whispers that I won't remember the next lyric or judges the way I have delivered a note. It's a constant battle.

## Lessons Learned

When I allow my Performer to lead, I am most grounded and can enjoy life. However, my Perfectionist does serve me by keeping me on top of all the details my life requires. And, I must acknowledge my Professional as the one who is best at keeping it together in difficult situations, and at making a nice presentation.

I want to expand on the idea of Gremlins. You will hear me refer to two of my biggest Gremlins regularly - The Perfectionist and the Rebel. Gremlin is a term that describes the inner voices that hates change and demands the status quo. They are the old tapes we continually play in our heads that attempt to keep us safe or make us small; the truth is that they often keep us from moving forward and getting what we want out of life. The goal is to recognize that these Gremlins (sorry to tell you that nearly everyone has several) are merely aspects of who we are. We need to be aware of their existence in order to stop the "knee-jerk reaction" that allows them take the driver's seat in our lives.

The key to *Stepping into More* is to empathize with each aspect of ourselves and to give each one a voice so that we can make a conscious choice in any given situation (a constant juggling act). My challenge is to catch myself in the moment, make a deliberate choice about which one will serve me best, and then to forgive myself when any one of them goes overboard. These may not be easy tasks but they are all part of my journey as a Recovering Perfectionist.

## Deepen Your Learning

1. **How do you define Perfectionism?**

   _____
   _____
   _____
   _____

2. Where do you see Perfectionism in your life? How does it impact your life?

   _____
   _____
   _____
   _____

3. What Gremlins are parts of your personality? How do you know when your Gremlins are in the driver's seat? What thoughts and feelings let you know your Gremlins are present? How do your Gremlins think they are serving you?

   _____
   _____
   _____
   _____

4. How do you define Performing for yourself? When are you on top of your game?

   _____
   _____
   _____
   _____

5. How do you know you are performing at your best? What do you notice about yourself? What types of thoughts, feelings, and physical sensations do you experience?

   _____
   _____
   _____
   _____

# 2
# A Star is Born

Junior high school was my time to start sharing my voice with the world. I asked my mom if I could take voice lessons and she allowed it, as long as I continued with my ballet and piano lessons. I love to dance but I really didn't want to be a prima ballerina like all the other girls in ballet class, and I had no discipline or desire to learn piano. I was in that pre-teen, chubby, awkward phase after getting my first period, and I felt lame and fat in my little pink skirt over my leotard. I would often cry to my voice teacher about my situation. All I wanted to do was sing! I was so adamant about not wanting to take ballet or piano that I forgot most of what I had learned.

My second voice teacher, the recently deceased Jack Halloran, was wonderful! I have such warm memories of singing along with the popular tracks on his cassette tapes (that was way before karaoke and CD tracks), and I loved the music we worked on – Barbara Streisand, Melissa Manchester, The Beatles. We also practiced vocal exercises (which wasn't nearly as much fun as singing pop songs). He gave me such encouragement and positive reinforcement.

My passion for singing was also rewarded when I began singing with the kids' choir at my synagogue. The Cantor was very supportive and asked me to sing a beautiful solo; he was so impressed that he actually took me to visit his own voice teacher. I began singing for the more than 800 people in the synagogue many Saturdays, which was a big deal. Beforehand, I was shaking and worrying that I might need water thinking about everything that could go wrong. But once I started singing, I felt a huge release from letting my voice soar. I felt the vibrato bubbling through every inch of me until it exploded out of my mouth. I was so connected to the feeling of the song even though it was in ancient Hebrew, which I didn't always understand or believe in, but that's a whole other story. My parents were also very proud that I was participating in the choir as they regularly attended services and felt a connection to the Jewish traditions.

The synagogue experience helped me build up enough confidence to start auditioning for school and camp plays, and I actually began landing great parts: I played Sandy in "Grease" and Peter in "Peter Pan" at my Jewish camp (I performed both plays entirely in Hebrew!). We called "Grease" "schmaltz" (Yiddish for "chicken fat"). Art started imitating life when I briefly dated the boy who played Danny in "Grease." People were intrigued by our hook up, but I quickly realized that I wasn't really attracted to him and broke things off.

The most challenging part of that play was when Sandy plays the tough girl at the end and sings, "You're the One That I Want." In tight jeans and heels, I was way out of my comfort zone. I was asked to strut my stuff in front of 500 campers. I was about to walk across the huge dining hall floor where we were performing feeling disgustingly fat and embarrassed to wear the skin tight jeans. I certainly didn't feel like I was exuding any sex appeal. In fact, I felt ridiculous. But it was fantastic to be heard and recognized by my peers. Even though I wasn't part of the popular clique, at least I was known for having a talent they respected.

I starred in school plays and more people began to recognize my talent. How I loved finding a sense of uniqueness! That was also when my crazy, rebellious side began to flourish. I loved doing goofy things, making people laugh, and being spontaneous. I would drink from the water fountain and then let the water stream out of my mouth and down my shirt. I made strange faces as I did it and many people found me quite entertaining.

I also developed some bad habits including a little bit of cheating in school (stemming from a fear of bad grades). Grades were everything to me because they were required in my household. If I didn't get good grades, I felt like I was failing life. After all, that was my big responsibility as a young adult and I had to perform. My family was big on showing one's intelligence and "being right." Good grades proved my intelligence and, therefore, made me a worthy person. Without the grades, I was a moron not worthy of existence (This was how I internalized things. This was not explicitly expressed by my parents). My quest for good grades caused me to do whatever it took: study hard and...cheat when all else failed.

I also experimented with alcohol during that time. I actually snuck into the synagogue's wine closet and stole bottles of wine (I only did it a couple of times!). I would also finish adults' half-empty glasses of wine. Part of me wanted to explode and go crazy while still meeting my parents' steep expectations. Drinking was a way to get out of my head and just be.

My first major audition was for my synagogue's production of "Fiddler on the Roof" at the age of 14. I auditioned with the song, "What I Did for Love" from "A Chorus Line." I climbed the stairs of the big stage and placed my battery operated cassette player on the floor to play the music track Mr. Halloran, my voice teacher recorded. I felt my voice quiver as I sang the first few lines. My arms literally fell asleep they were so tight. My voice was alive but my body was practically dead. As I entered the chorus, I felt my confidence rising and my voice became more certain. I ended with a long, impressive note and received applause. Despite my jittery nerves, I sang very well. Unfortunately I knew that my acting audition wasn't as strong, but they wound up creating two additional younger-daughter parts – one for me, and the other for my soon to be older friend, Eydie.

I had so many mixed emotions during the production: I was thrilled to be in a pretty serious production *and* I felt like I should have more visibility and lines. I actually resented not having a bigger part. A girl who was a year older got the lead role that I wanted. Man, was I jealous! I practically lost my voice during every performance in my determination to be heard during the large group numbers.

It was at this time that I started experimenting with drugs. I took a Quaalude for the first time during our cast party. I sat on the couch looking around me and despite my best efforts, I couldn't remember what anyone was saying and my head was spinning. I kept asking

*"What did you say?"* for most of the evening.

I took that drug one other time after the cast party before completing a homework assignment. Miraculously, I was able to write a paper while under the influence. There was such a push/pull going on in my soul between my two Gremlins - the Perfectionist and my adolescent Rebel. I longed to break free from the many rules in my world and, yet, I still had the sense that I should live up to the many expectations placed on me. I really focused on doing well in school, and becoming a more diligent student. As long as I got good grades, I figured I could pretty much get away with anything else.

But I got taken down a notch while participating in the making of a Jewish music record with Craig P., an up-and-coming Jewish recording artist. We were a group of high school kids making a record of Jewish songs in a mix of Hebrew and English, and performing at various venues. Along with many of my friends from the choir, I auditioned for at least six solo songs. Craig praised my vocal ability a lot, and yet I wasn't chosen to sing even one of the solos. I was so jealous and angry because some of my friends who didn't sing well at all did get solos.

But what a thrill it was to record a record! I put on the studio headsets and I felt like I was on a mission from God to be heard on this album (even without a solo). Again, I practically lost my voice from belting out my parts so I could be heard. When I listened to the final product, I felt great pride because no one could deny that I was a big part of the record. And then, Craig asked me to sing, "The Star Spangled Banner" at our live performances. It wasn't a recording —

and I was embarrassed and grateful at the same time — but at least I finally had my solo.

The record experience was bittersweet as it would result in my disconnecting from several friends who were on the project. My jealousy because I didn't get a solo on the record or during our live performances played a part in this, I can now say, some 26 years later.

But high school was an interesting time; I was a strange creature who hadn't found her home. I was enrolled in many advanced classes – except for math. Around that time, I learned that I had blanked out on about four years of math during junior high school. My grandfather was a mathematician and not the nicest of individuals. I remember his quizzing me in math during kindergarten and screaming,

*"What is five plus five?"*

I gave some sort of response.

*"No! It's ten!"*

That was one of my first experiences with the pressure to perform on demand. My grandfather had traumatized me so much that I completely blanked out four years of math. I was struggling terribly in my high school math class and my mother thought a hypnotist could help me improve my grades. One of the first things he did was to test my IQ. I don't know how accurate his process was (since he coached me through some of the responses), but he told me that I was quite bright. During the hypnotherapy sessions, he would have me lay in a reclining chair while he spoke calmly and softly and played some sort of tapes. I don't know how helpful it was since I would usually fall asleep. He would say,

*"Don't worry. Your subconscious picked up everything you needed to know."*

I felt like I had flunked Hypnotherapy 101. I also was awarded my first (and only) "D" in Geometry. My Perfectionist was quite embarrassed, ashamed, and humiliated. I had studied my ass off, met with the teacher after school, worked with a tutor, and had gone to a hypnotist, and I still sucked.

Years later, I ran into my math teacher, Mr. White. He told me that he couldn't remember what grade I had gotten in his class but that I was a very diligent student who had tried very hard. That was gratifying. I had accepted my fate – I am terrible at math – but somehow, I was still able to leave my house each morning. I felt shame over having such an imperfection but, on the flip side, I felt okay about having done my best.

High school was also the time that I entered into "play production," which was amazing. We performed at Shakespeare festivals, as well as in school plays. I really loved performing and I managed to get out of my head and start improvising. At one school performance, some fellow students were trying to warm up the crowd before a play and I jumped onto the stage and started doing and saying wacky things. I didn't know what I was going to do or say. I felt an incredible surge of adrenalin and the desire to be seen and to make people laugh. Guess what: people actually laughed! Just "going for it" without a plan was such a great feeling. I loved standing out and having people notice me. Finally, I wasn't invisible.

But I reached the pinnacle of my identity crisis between my Perfectionist and Rebel when I decided to shave three stripes on either side of my head. I felt like I didn't fit in anywhere so I might as well stand out. I had thought about taking this daring step for awhile and finally decided to do it the day of my boyfriend's prom. It seemed like a special occasion to do something out of the box. My hairdresser Demetri was very excited to give me such an unusual haircut. He said it would have been better if he had been under the influence of something but, alas, he had to complete his mission sober (as far as I know). He put the finishing touches on my special "do" by putting red mousse in my hair. I looked like an art piece. I was excited by my new look and nervous as hell. Shaving my head was a bold statement for me (although I'm not quite sure what the message was). I had never done anything so radical before and I had the sense of, "I'll show 'em" (whoever "they" might've been).

I felt so bad for my boyfriend when I arrived in my beautiful, blue, formal dress and my really strange red hairstyle. He didn't react too strongly (he was in love with me no matter what), and I was a bit surprised that he wasn't turned off by my "new look." His mom actually told me she liked my "punky" style.

During dinner, my boyfriend's friend came up to our table and asked,

*"Did you know your date has a Mohawk?"*

I thought I was going to die of embarrassment. I was being seen alright, but not in the way I truly wanted to be noticed.

After the dance, we drove with another couple to a street from which you could see the airport runway. He wanted to make out but I was angry and not feeling connected to him (and probably more importantly, not very much to myself, either). Poor guy, I broke up with him that night. I couldn't stand being with him when I was feeling so much distance from him and most especially from myself. Instead of spending the night at his parents' house (in a separate room, of course), I went home early. My mom came into my room in the morning, looked at me, and said,

*"You are so ugly"* and promptly closed the door.

Those words stung and I felt the tears flowing.

It was a very awkward time. I wore preppy clothing for the most part – Polo shirts, Levi's and Topsider shoes. So there I was – this preppy-dressed girl with punk stripes on her head taking advanced-level classes and hanging out with wacky kids from the play-production group. I was a sight! I would walk around school and the punkers would look at me like, "Who the hell is this strange-looking chick?" I attended my honor-level classes with the cliques of girls who seemed to be thinking, "What happened to Rachel? She is so strange." Many of the play-production kids were doing a lot of drugs in their quest to be different and experience life. I didn't feel like I quite fit in with them either, as much as I wanted to. I couldn't wait for my hair to grow back. I decided that I didn't like that type of attention. I felt like a freak.

That was also the time that my dad decided to move to Boston for yet another business opportunity. My mom was adamant that she didn't want to move and stayed with my brother and me in Los Angeles. Our family listened to Peter Allen's "Bi-Coastal" record a lot during that time. On my first visit to Boston, my dad saw my hair but didn't have much of a reaction. I don't think he wanted me to know how freaked out he was. Now, my mom was resorting to using reverse-psychology on me. She encouraged me to buy thrift-store clothes to better suit my hairstyle (interesting approach!). I actually did go to Aardvark's thrift shop in Hollywood with a friend and bought a very cute "puke green" summer dress. I wore it with pink high-heeled shoes. I ditched school one day and went to Denny's in Hollywood with my friend Susan and overheard this old lady whispering to her friend,

*"Look at that punker."*

I felt funny, uncomfortable and strange. I certainly wasn't a punker but I didn't know who or what I was.

High school was a time of experimentation – you name it, I experimented with it. My parents laid low as long as I got good grades. I was definitely pushing the limits and having so much fun. Somehow, I was keeping it all together.

The fact that I wasn't getting as many lead roles as I would have liked in play production was frustrating, but it didn't stop me from having quite an adventure. Being part of the group and collaboratively creating meant a lot to me. Now truly a part of a creative community, I had many good friends and good times.

After a while, the bi-coastal thing wasn't working so well for my parents; my dad wanted a divorce. At a crucial point, I went with my mom to the airport so she could try to persuade him to change his mind. She was on a mission to save the marriage, and whatever she did worked. She finally agreed to move to Boston. I was soooo sick of moving. At that point, I was about to begin my senior year and I had no desire to move again. A friend of mine was planning to go to the American Academy of Dramatic Arts, so I gathered the courage to ask my parents about attending. To my surprise, my dad actually agreed. I was truly shocked.

My plans were to graduate high school a semester early and then attend the academy (assuming I was accepted). My parents legally emancipated me during my semester-long senior year so that they could move to Boston. I remember coming in late and then signing my own late notes – a teenager's dream come true! During that semester, I was living in my parent's amazing condo and I had so much fun there. I did just enough to get by in school. I also got to direct a piece for a competition in play production. My Performer was sprung free and was playing and experimenting. I felt very proud even though we didn't win anything. That was the most free I had ever felt.

**Lessons Learned**

Junior High School and High School was an awkward time filled with much angst and great discovery. This was when I unearthed my innate ability to self-express through my voice. I learned that I was able to be seen and heard in a positive way when I was singing and performing. This was also the time that my competitiveness surfaced. I competed with others and mostly with myself. I needed to be in the spotlight both on stage and in the classroom. My Perfectionist was driving me to be successful at almost any cost. It didn't matter if I cheated in school or hurt friends – I needed to come out on top to prove my worthiness as a human being. This was also when my Rebel stood out front and center. I yearned to let loose from the long list of expectations placed on me by myself and others. My Rebel resents these expectations and sometimes engages in unhealthy behavior in an attempt to escape and be free my Perfectionist's never ending demands. To this day, I experience the push/pull between my Perfectionist and my Rebel.

**Deepen Your Learning**

1. How do you self-express? What means do you prefer?

   _____
   _____
   _____
   _____

2. Are you competitive? If yes, what drives your competitiveness? How do you feel inside when you are competitive? What behaviors do you engage in when you are competitive? How do these behaviors serve and/or hurt you?

   _____
   _____
   _____
   _____

3. How realistic are the expectations that you place on yourself? What can you do to modify expectations if they aren't realistic?

   _____
   _____
   _____
   _____

4. Do you have an inner Rebel? What does he/she look and feel like? What behaviors do you in engage in when your Rebel is at play? How does your Rebel think he/she is serving you? How does your Rebel serve and/or hurt you?

   _____
   _____
   _____
   _____
   _____

5. How do you balance your desire to be successful while still feeling free and joyous?

   _____
   _____
   _____
   _____
   _____

# 3
## From Method Acting to Singing Telegram

The time had come for me to attend the American Academy of Dramatic Arts. My friend had started one semester before me and found an apartment for us to share. Unfortunately, the apartment was small, I had to share a room with my friend who was a major slob, and the building was located in the middle of hell! When my boyfriend dropped me off there after a date, I remember sitting in his car not wanting to go upstairs. I was scared to walk in; the sound of ambulance and police-car sirens was non-stop. It didn't take long for me to decide to move back into my parents' vacant luxurious condo despite the long drive to and from Pasadena — I had my priorities straight!

Acting school had its highs and lows. As the youngest student enrolled at the time, I was intimidated and continually felt like I had to prove myself. But with a variety of acting, voice and movement classes, the program was exciting and it stretched me on many levels. I learned that I could actually dance! I enjoyed moving my body to the music. My confidence began building, as well. For a mock audition in one of my classes, I even went out and bought a shiny silver bodysuit (how '80s!) that definitely showed off my curves. That was a definite stretch for me since I normally tried to hide my body. We learned and auditioned choreography to a Stray Cats song and, much to my surprise, I got a callback for another round of auditions! That was when my nerves kicked in; I was so uptight that I stumbled through the second audition and didn't "get the part."

At first, I loved the acting classes. We went through sensory exercises such as imagining we were first very hot and then very cold. One time, I was so into an activity that I began to shiver from imagining being in the snow. When I was assigned my first kissing scene, I didn't know how to handle it. My partner Tad was a nice guy who happened to be gay. I was so nervous that I instinctively stuck my tongue in his mouth during our kiss (a very awkward moment!). He stared at me in shock. I think my class was stunned as well as they sat in silence. It was the beginning of the big AIDS scare and I was nervous that I might become infected. In those early days, no one knew how it was transmitted and a lot of misinformation was bandied about. Thankfully, I remained healthy – just a bit embarrassed.

During one of the plays, I was assigned to play a "hippy" character that blew bubbles mostly from underneath a table. I only had few lines. I got really into the character and practiced blowing bubbles and zoning out so much that I literally felt like I was under the influence. That was fun.

But the acting became increasingly painful for me. I enjoy acting as a release to get in touch with emotions and out of my head. I was introduced to "Method Acting" and Uta Hagen's approach. I was instructed to attach a real-life memory to practically every moment in the script. It was an approach that took me straight into my Perfectionist head. I got so caught up in doing it "right" that I had difficulty "feeling" the character. My instructors had become increasingly critical and I felt very disconnected. I now know that there are many approaches to acting, and that those that involve focusing on being "in the moment" fit me much better. But at the time, I just felt like I was failing and disappointing my teachers.

I was even struggling in my voice class. This was hard for me to take as one of the few things in life I was certain about is that I had a good voice. Mr. Peck, our vocal teacher assigned me some very challenging songs. The first song he tasked me with singing was

"Memories" from the musical Cats. I had been preparing for over one week. I learned the lyrics and my pitch and vibrato were perfect. I was nervous as this was my first performance in front of the class and this was a difficult song. Nonetheless, I was expecting praise because I knew I could sing.

Class started and my classmates began performing. Some were awful which made me feel more at ease. Some sounded amazing which scared me. I sat, fidgeting in my chair in anticipation of my turn. Finally my turn arrived. I timidly approached the center of the room, stood in front of my teacher and classmates and signaled to the piano player to begin. I belted the song, feeling the vibrato bubble deep inside me and shoot out my mouth like a fire hose filled with energy, enveloping the room. I was so nervous that I barely moved my body. I held the last note for what felt like an eternity, finished, and awaited my undoubtedly glowing feedback.

Instead, Mr. Peck told me

*"I want you to sing with more meaning. Sing from your heart."*

I was dumbfounded and shocked! I felt like I was pouring my entire being into the song but Mr. Peck wanted me to give more. I wasn't sure what else I could bring. I sang the song again determined to please him and yet, once again received a similar response. I didn't get it. What did he want from me?!

The next song he assigned was "Crossword Puzzle" from Starting Here, Starting Now, and it kicked my butt! It's a Sondheim story-song with a million lyrics; I was struggling just to understand and remember the lyrics, never mind convey the story. To make matters worse, he wanted me to limit my vibrato! That is a skill I have always been proud of and it was hard for me to control it.

I decided I wanted to make money from my singing so I auditioned for a singing-telegram job with Eastern Onion (I lied and told them I was 18). I declined when they asked me if I wanted to be a stripper, but told them I would be happy to be an opening act for the strippers. The job turned out to be quite different than I had anticipated. They provided a huge book with hundreds of songs, tapes of all the songs, and a leash – in other words, a pager. I had three costumes in my trunk ready to be called into action at a moment's notice: The "French Onion Maid," "The Giant Heart" and, my personal favorite, "The Layer Cake with a Cherry on Top" (in the form of a red cherry hat)!

I was sitting in acting class one day when suddenly, I received a page from Eastern Onion. I excused myself, found a pay phone (that was before cell phones) and called.

*"Song 23b, cake outfit, in Van Nuys — can you make it in two hours?"*
*"Hell no,"* I said. *"I'm in the middle of class!"*

Once, I was sent to sing a "get well" song for a patient at UCLA hospital. The song was about how much they were loved and cared for but I blanked out in the middle of the song and sang,

*"...and if you don't get well...nobody cares!"*

On another adventure, they sent me to the gang-ridden Watts section of Los Angeles in the sexy French Maid costume. There I was, 17 years old, driving by myself in the middle of a scary neighborhood looking for the right house (some of which were tin shacks covered with graffiti). I found the house and knocked on the door when a strange woman opened the door staring at me with surprise. Wrong house! Finally, I came to the right house and was greeted by a bunch of Latino people who didn't understand English!

The worst part about that job was that I made practically no money. They paid $10-$15 per gig, and I rarely got tips because the telegrams were pricey. They didn't even pay for all my mileage. A couple of times, I was the opening act for a stripper. I did my act with my clapping wind-up monkey, sang a little and then welcomed the stripper. It was a strange environment for a girl like me but at least they only went topless and there wasn't any lap dancing (ha!).

The final straw on that job was the time I was with a friend enjoying lunch at a restaurant in Pasadena and the leash went off. I found a pay phone and was told:

*"Song 54, the cake outfit in Upland. You need to be there in one hour."*

That was going to be a challenge since I had no idea where Upland was (I only knew that it was far away!) and I had no clue how to sing - Song 54. GPS devices had not yet been invented so I pulled out my map book and started navigating. I abruptly finished lunch, got changed, and started driving while frantically learning Song 54. I was so nervous that my stomach was in knots, and I had no idea where I was driving.

*Why am I doing this?*

I kept asking myself. By the time I arrived, I was so panicked that I wrote the words down on a piece of paper. I performed my opening number without a problem using my mechanical monkey as a prop. But as I was about to sing the telegram, I realized that I forgot not only the lyrics but also the melody! I reached underneath my cake outfit to find the lyrics I had tucked into my tights. I read the telegram without much emotion. I was completely embarrassed and ashamed. That was my last gig. Enough was enough. This was too stressful and not worth the aggravation. Yet, the Perfectionist in me was disappointed that I couldn't make this job work and that somehow I had failed.

By the end of that year, I was frustrated, nervous, and insecure. I had some successes but felt like I was behind the eight ball and not talented enough. I was shocked when I opened the form letter from the Academy informing me that I had not been accepted into their second-year program. I was caught off guard and then suddenly every bit of negative feedback that I received during the last year flashed in front of my face. All the pieces seemed to come together. I didn't realize the feedback was severe enough to warrant me not being accepted. I couldn't believe it!

I scheduled an appointment to speak with the principal but meeting with him didn't change my status. Later, a fellow student informed me that if I had written a letter requesting to be accepted, they would have let me in (it had happened to her and her acting ability was certainly no better than mine).

That was my first big REJECTION!!! I was devastated and embarrassed. I felt like a huge failure. I told myself,

*You obviously suck at this, so it's time to move on with your life and do something practical.*

I was so insecure that I decided my first rejection would be my last. I couldn't take the humiliation. I worked for my dad's check-cashing store for a brief stint (and I have plenty of stories to tell about that experience); within six months, I was enrolled at California State University, Northridge. Without consciously knowing it, I had just shut the door on my creativity for the next 23 years.

During my first semester at California State University, Northridge, I was a Psychology major because I always had a knack for helping family and friends with their problems. But I quickly realized that I had no desire to work with clinically mental ill people. Frankly, it scared me. My second semester, I decided to be very practical by changing my major to Business Administration with an emphasis in Human Resources Management. I thought my parents would think this was a respectable degree that could potentially lead me to a *normal career*.

**Lessons Learned**

Acting school was bittersweet for me. In the beginning, I trusted my talent and abilities. I also experienced incredible freedom living on my own for the first time. I started tapping into my ability to feel the fear and do it anyway. My perfectionism quickly took over and I doubted my abilities to perform both in school and as a singing telegram. I quickly retreated and let my Perfectionist lead me to the more traditional college route. Looking back, I realized that too much structure takes me out of the "being" of the creative process and this is when my perfectionism kicks in. Even as an adult I struggle with how to truly allow my creativity to surface without turning it into a work project that I need to accomplish and conquer.

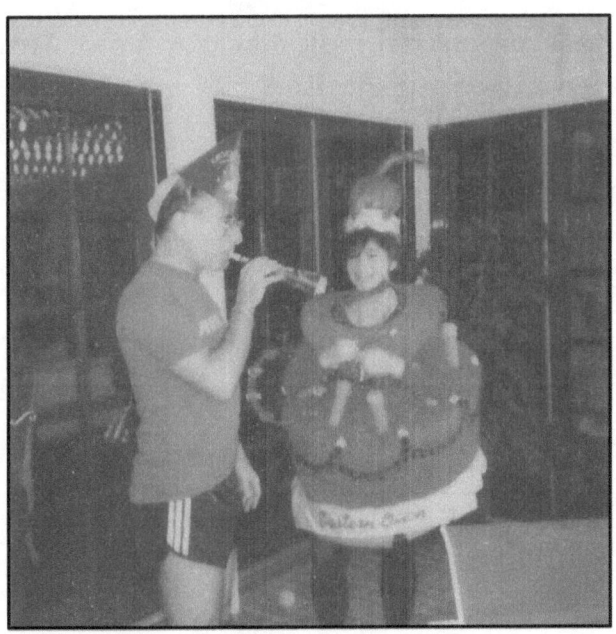

**Deepen Your Learning**

1. **What is a life rule that you believe and abide by? How does this rule serve and/or hinder you?**

   _____
   _____
   _____
   _____

2. What frightens you? Where do these fears originate? How much of your fears are based on fact and reality?

3. What does creativity look like for you? How do you express creativity in your life?

4. How could you bring more creativity into your life?

5. Describe a big rejection you experienced? How did you handle it? What did you learn from the experience?

# 4
# Two Weddings and a Business Degree

My parents were shocked when I told them I was going to be a business major:

*"How are you going to be able to pass all the math and accounting classes?"* they asked.

Good question... how ironic that they would plant seeds of doubt in my head just as I was embarking on a "practical" career. But their lack of confidence somehow increased my determination to get through the program. Amazingly, I survived three accounting, two statistics, two economics and one finance class. Guess what? I disliked them all and really struggled, but I studied my ass off and did (almost) whatever it took to succeed. The stakes were high since most of my identity was tied to my getting good grades.

I was so relieved when I took my first management development class and fell in love with it. We were talking about motivation, communication and employee development. I knew very quickly that this was where I fit into the corporate world puzzle. I also took Human Resources classes; I wasn't passionate about the tactical components but I was excited about the human elements. I also didn't quite understand how that "softer side" of business would be accepted in the real world. Immediately after discovering the "feminine" part of business, doubt and fear settled in. I wondered how a "sensitive" woman like me would make it in the corporate arena? How would I fit into the "man's business world"?

My singing pretty much took a nosedive during my four and a half years of college. In fact, my only memory of sharing my voice was while recording an answering machine message to my parody of the Beatles tune, "Let It Be," which went something like this:

*When I find myself sitting on the toilet*
*And I hear the phone ring*
*I thank Mother Mary my machine is on.*
*I can't let it ring.*
*Let it ring, let it ring, let it ring, let it ring.*
*I'm currently incapacitated,*
*So let it ring!*

I joined a supposedly co-ed business fraternity (it was really just a bunch of wild party animals), and during my initiation weekend, I was blindfolded and led into a dark room with glaring interrogation lights and crowds of people surrounding me. The head hazer told me how disappointed he was with my telephone message and how unprofessional it was. The crowd started to boo and hiss. Wow – this was scary and uncomfortable! Then he asked me to sing my telephone greeting for everyone; people were laughing and screaming out obscenities. It was quite a moment! I was conflicted and confused. Of course, I knew that hazing was supposed to be a little cruel. But with my insecurities about my voice, I didn't really know if they liked my singing or not, and I felt a bit ashamed that I had recorded such an unprofessional song. But I acted tough and laughed along.

Being in that fraternity was an interesting experience, which highlights a theme in the way that I "show up." Part of me desperately wanted to be accepted and be part of the gang. I wanted to know that I was included. Yet there was another part of me that was a bit of a loner.

There are times when I want to be my own person and don't want to feel obligated to go to events or hang with certain people. Other times I can feel excluded and a bit of an outsider. I now own the fact that sometimes, I have been the one who excluded me. That is a pattern that continues to this day making me wonder:

*How can I fit in and still remain my own person?*
*How can I be part of a community, but on my own terms?*

College was also the time that I got married – can you believe it?! I was only 21! I had met my Ron (my husband of more than 23 years) in Israel when I was 13 and he was 15. It was a wonderful twist of fate because our parents had met seven or eight years prior through mutual friends when they lived in Los Angeles briefly. We had never met while they were in Los Angeles. After my Bat-Mitzvah, we met for the first time and hung out together in Israel. When I was 16, I went back again on a group trip and we had a "fling." I felt guilty as I was cheating on my boyfriend of two weeks from the group trip, but I really liked Ron. I even wrote in my journal:

*It's too bad he lives so far away because he is so nice.*

Upon my return, I wrote to him but I didn't hear back. Oh well...

When I was 20, my best friend Daphne and I decided to go to Israel for the summer. I wrote Ron a letter and, to my surprise, his younger brother Gil (who recently tragically passed away from a brain aneurism at the age of 45) answered me with a surprisingly flirtatious letter. When we arrived in Israel, we double dated with Ron and Gil for one week. One evening, we went to a large disco. I was dancing with Gil while the U2 song "Sunday Bloody Sunday" was playing. In the middle of the dance he left the dance floor for no apparent reason. I was confused and felt like a loser. Later we were hanging out in their old, white Volkswagen van outside Daphne's cousin's house. Ron and Daphne almost kissed, and I almost kissed Gil. But I had a burning feeling that I didn't want Daphne near Ron. I suddenly realized that I had feelings for Ron and I needed to show him quickly before the summer went in a whole other direction.

When we returned home that evening, I told Daphne that I still liked Ron after all these years. We made the following pact:

*"Whatever happens on our date the next night...happens."*

To me, that meant: I would make Ron mine, and I was determined to make it so.

That next night, we hung out at Ron and Gil's house; I was on a mission from God to claim Ron. My intention was clear – I needed to outlast everyone until Ron and I could be alone. At around 11:00 p.m. I was still crazy hyper, full of energy, but both Gil and Daphne were dozing off. Gil said goodnight and went to his room to sleep. While Gil was trying to sleep, I started sneaking in his room to wake him up. I did this to get Ron's attention. But every time I got near Gil's door, Ron stopped me from entering. Both of us became more aggressive; I wanted in and Ron was guarding the door. He grabbed my arms trying to stop me and then suddenly, there was a sexual feeling to his touch. I was very excited. I finally burst into Gil's room with Ron still holding on to me and managed to wake Gil up. When he opened his eyes, he saw Ron's body slammed against mine, holding me around the waist from behind. I was sure he could feel the romantic tension when he looked at us with a surprised and amused look.

When Ron dropped Daphne and me off at her cousin's apartment building later that evening, Daphne went upstairs and Ron and I finally stood alone. We looked awkwardly at each other until he kissed me. I could feel my heart pounding and the excitement rushing through my veins. It was a quick kiss but it was enough to know that he was mine, and I his. Mission accomplished! I later found out that he had had the same talk with Gil the night before to tell him that he was interested in me. At the time, I felt like my intentional fight to win Ron over had worked. Now I know that our relationship was meant to be.

We dated that summer and it was the best summer and time of my life. I was young, skinny and pretty. Many Israelis like being around American girls (especially men), and they were very complimentary. Ron and I went on numerous dates and were very into each other. I remember getting ready for our dates – I was so excited; I couldn't wait for the privilege of being alone with this special man. Oh, the long and joyful "make out" sessions in his parents' white Volkswagen van! We could kiss for hours! When it came time to go home, I was very depressed and didn't want to leave.

We corresponded for a semester and it was painful not being with him so I decided to return to Tel Aviv University for the following semester. I had the sneaky suspicion that Ron was "the one," so I started dating like crazy to get it out of my system. I dated others casually during our semester apart and for some reason I suddenly became very popular with the boys. I told them up front I was going to Israel to be with Ron and that seemed to attract them more; one even gave me a necklace. Perhaps I had become more desirable because I appeared to be more of a conquest.

I remember boarding the plane to Israel to embark on my semester long journey. I was blasting Steve Miller's "Big Ol Jet Airliner" as the plane took off. Tears rolled down my cheek as I realized life would probably never be the same. On our first night together upon my return to Israel, we lay in his room listening to Pink Floyd's "Dark Side of the Moon." The moment I had been waiting for (for months) had finally arrived. We connected both physically and emotionally; it was a wonderful beginning.

Our bond continued to grow during my trip. I never felt as free as a person and I loved every minute we spent together. As the semester continued, I had this nagging fear about the future. I didn't want our time together to end. What did the future hold?

Ron finished his obligatory military service at the same time that I completed my semester. I begged him to join me on a trip to Europe but he chose to go on a safari adventure in South America with his friend instead. I was devastated.

The night before we went our separate ways, we had a date on the beach in Tel Aviv. The sun was setting and we sat on the sand watching the day turn into night. I had prepared a special song for him – James Taylor's "Close Your Eyes." Such fitting lyrics –

*"Well, the sun is slowly sinking down, the moon is surely rising. This old world must still be spinning round, and I still love you!*

*So close your eyes. You can close your eyes it's alright. I don't know no love songs. I can't sing the blues anymore, but I can sing this song, and you can sing this song when I'm gone!"*

I was sad and angry. How could he choose his friend over me? What was he thinking? What was going to happen to our beautiful relationship? We parted ways and I was devastated.

On the Fourth of July, I called home from Nice, France where I was traveling with a wonderful guy friend. Luckily, there was no physical attraction between us and he had been a total gentleman. When I spoke to my mom, she said,

*"You will never guess who's visiting the U.S."*

It was Ron!

I was shocked and confused. Ron later told me that he was nearly kidnapped in Ecuador and that they decided to fly to Miami, buy an old station wagon and drive across America to California. By the time I stepped off the plane in Los Angeles, Ron was there to pick me up. It was like a dream come true!

My parents were living in New York and, initially, they said that Ron had to find a separate apartment and that I had to live with my brother Adam while he completed his senior year of high school. My brother was 17 going on 12; he was extremely rebellious and was drinking and doing drugs. To put it mildly, I was not excited about moving in with him. I told my parents that one of two things would happen if Ron got his own apartment:

1) I would stay at Ron's place regularly and we would hardly see my brother

Or:

2) Ron would practically live at our apartment and I would lie about it

"So, which option do you prefer?" I asked them.

To my shock and amazement, they agreed that Ron could move in with Adam and me. We lived together for about six months, but it was definitely not like the show, "Three's Company." At the age of 21, I had been suddenly cast into a parental role while experiencing my first romantic live in situation. I wasn't ready for it and my brother resented it. My Perfectionist tried to get him to adhere to rules. At the same time my Rebel was at play and I wanted to be free. This was my first time living with a man. I was conflicted and it was an uncomfortable position to be in. My relationship with Adam has never been the same since.

Meanwhile, Ron's work visa expired and he was working illegally. It was clear that he would have to return to Israel unless he found a way to get a work permit; the only way for him to get a permit was for us to get married! I certainly hadn't envisioned myself marrying at such an early age, and it was a tough decision.

Ron was on the phone with his mom in Israel one day when I heard him say:

*"By the way, we might get married, but don't worry, it's no big deal and you don't need to come. If things don't work out, we can always get divorced."*

I am sure his mother must have been terrified. Actually, it shocked me, too. I was wondering:

*Was he ready to make a commitment?*
*Did he really love me?*

It's nice to have an "exit strategy," but the fact that we could "always get divorced" wasn't very comforting! He hung up the phone and asked me:

*"So, do you want to get hitched?"*

I told Ron that if he really wanted to get married, I needed a proper proposal.

*"What do you mean?"* he asked, a little baffled.

I told him that I wanted him to pick a restaurant and really ask me to marry him. With his eyes wide in confusion, he asked,

*"Okay, so...where do you want to eat?"*

I told him that he should take his time and find the restaurant himself. Being new to the country, he asked around in search of the right place. He found a wonderful restaurant, Chianti on Melrose Avenue. It was softly lit, Italian, and romantic.

We were both so nervous that we each drank a bottle of wine! As the evening went on, the anticipation built as I waited for the moment he would propose. Finally, Ron got down on one knee beside me and I gasped slightly knowing that this special moment had arrived.

As he looked at me with loving eyes, he asked,

*"Would you marry me?"*

It wasn't exactly the way I had imagined my engagement would be (everything was chaotic and a bit messy and there wasn't a ring), but deep down, I felt that Ron was authentic and that I was making a good choice. I was following my intuition since I was too young to be able to base my decision on experience. I let my perfectionism go out the window and listened to my heart.

Very moved, I took a breath and softly replied,

*"Yes!"*

At that point, we were both teary eyed. He stayed on his knee for a few moments before admitting,

*"I can't get up after all that wine."*

I had to assist him in getting to his feet. And then Ron told the waiter,

*"We're getting married!"*

The waiter announced our engagement to all the other restaurant patrons, and everyone clapped. I was going on trust and intuition. Everything about the situation was unconventional and I loved it!

Not too long thereafter, we arranged to have our wedding with "Reverend Bob" on a Sunday afternoon. We actually found him in the yellow pages. We decided not to wed with a Rabbi since, ultimately, we wanted to have a Jewish ceremony in Israel and you cannot be married twice by a Rabbi. My parents were mortified.

My mother sat me down and asked,

*"How can you marry him? He doesn't have any money."*

So I inquired,

*"Did dad have any money when you got married?"*

*"No,"* she admitted.

Then I said,

*"Well, things seemed to work out alright didn't they?"*

That seemed to settle the matter.

I decided to make the event as "wedding like" as possible, and went to Nordstrom where I found a simple and beautiful off-white dress. It wasn't a wedding dress; it was knee-length with long sleeves, and was quietly lovely and pretty. We invited about 20 of our friends; Ron's mother flew in from Israel, and his brother Gil (the one I had almost kissed many years before) came from Rhode Island where he was studying culinary arts. Even my old boyfriend who I had cheated on with Ron during my trip to Israel came.

The day of the wedding, we had no water in our apartment building; they were doing work on the building and it had been going on for days. It was so bad that we carried water from the fountain outside in order to flush the toilet! I rushed over to my friend Daphne's house (who had almost kissed Ron years ago) so I could at least take a shower before my wedding.

Despite that little setback, it actually turned out to be a lovely civil service at Reverend Bob's home. Our guests threw rice at us as we left the service (very un-Jewish). My parents treated all of us to a very nice lunch, and it all seemed to work. I was so in love with Ron that I got over the fact that I was taking the road less travelled. In fact, it was fun being different. The next day, I went to school and attended a business-fraternity meeting. As we went around the room sharing what we had done over the weekend, I stated,

*"I got married."*

Everyone was in shock. I was a bit shocked, myself!

Eleven months later in Israel, we had a huge wedding with about 375 guests, most of whom I didn't know. Unexpectedly, someone called me onto the stage and asked me to sing — I was mortified! I wasn't prepared and was shaking with fear. It upset me that I hadn't been told I would be singing, but part of me was excited by the opportunity.

I decided to sing, "Memory" from "Cats" and the band did its best to follow me. I was so nervous that I forgot some of the words, but I carried on and hit all the notes. I have no clue as to how I sounded; I was just relieved to have survived the experience.

My parents and I still disagree about which wedding date counts, and about the number of years that Ron and I have been married. Ron and I celebrate on the date of our second wedding, but add one year in honor of the first wedding. Or, we will tell people something like:

*"We've been married for 22/23 years."*

It can be very confusing for people.

The first years of our marriage were fun and carefree. Ron and I moved into a new apartment (without my brother). It was so much fun having our own place, our own schedules, and doing whatever we pleased. All was good until I was about to graduate college. I was lying in bed with Ron (who was hoping to get lucky that morning) thinking about the future when, suddenly, an enormous weight settled on my shoulders and in my heart. I realized that I was now a married woman who was about to be thrust into a career and had to be able to support herself. I was still in my early twenties, but my parents were planning to stop supporting us as soon as I graduated from college! The weight and pressure of those thoughts all but killed my sex drive for years. From that day forward, I felt I was under tremendous pressure to deliver the goods (I wasn't talking about sexual goods) if we were going to survive.

**Lessons Learned**

College turned out different than I planned. I could never have predicted falling in love with an Israeli, getting married and living with my brother. College was a time that I proved to myself I could accomplish challenges despite my fears as long as I put my mind to it. I noticed that I was conflicted by wanting to be accepted and validated by others while still being able to set boundaries. I learned to be more assertive with my parents - ask for what I needed and speak my truth. I also learned the beauty of listening to my heart and following my intuition. I made one of the best decisions of my life – to marry my husband just by trusting my gut. This was a time where I also strayed from my love of singing and performing. Although I was gratified to discover my avocation, a part of me was longing to find the courage and avenue to bring singing back into my life.

## Deepen Your Learning

1. Have you ever abandoned your dreams? What was the impact? What got in your way?

   _____
   _____
   _____
   _____

2. How important is it for you to be liked and receive external validation from others? How does this impact what actions you take and decisions you make?

   _____
   _____
   _____
   _____

3. Think back to a time that you followed your intuition? What was the result of your decision? What did you learn about yourself?

   _____
   _____
   _____
   _____

4. How comfortable are you speaking your truth and asking for what you want? How can this benefit you? What is the impact when you don't?

   _____
   _____
   _____
   _____

# 5
## I Dreamed a Dream

I didn't sing with any regularity for many years. I felt like it was too late and that I wasn't talented enough. Now 21 years old and in business school, my Perfectionist told me that it was either black or white: since I couldn't fulfill my original vision, I had to let it go and move on. Still, I couldn't let go of singing completely. I felt like I was in mourning; I was mourning the loss of my creative, emotional self. I would go to plays and concerts and visualize myself on the stage, sharing my heart. I would literally cry, thinking about how this could have been *my* life. It took a lot of mental energy for me to keep processing all of it in my overloaded head. Alas, I conceded, my dream wasn't meant to be.

Over the next 24 years, I made wimpy unsuccessful attempts to step back into my creativity. Part of me wanted to sing, but I had become petrified of sharing my voice, of being vulnerable; and of the chance that someone might tell me I wasn't good enough. Conversely, another fear was that once people knew of my talent, they would obligate me to sing on demand. That reminded me way too much of my childhood; I still I don't like people telling me what to do and pressuring me to share my talent.

Not long after our first wedding, I was singing at my grandparents' fiftieth anniversary in Florida wearing the same pretty dress I had worn to my wedding (at least I got good use out of the dress!). My grandma asked me to sing something in Hebrew, and I decided on an excerpt from a prayer that I used to sing in synagogue with a beautiful, unique melody that showed off my voice. I had not sung that song since I was 12 when I was in the synagogue choir. I nervously awaited my turn to sing while one of my distant cousins sang "Memory" from "Cats." Despite his odd appearance, he really had a lovely voice, and I thought about all the songs I could have picked but hadn't. Then, I realized that I couldn't remember all the words to my Hebrew prayer. Now, I was really nervous!

My turn arrived and I took center stage on the dance floor surrounded by hundreds of people. I began singing with my hands glued to my sides. I felt so happy to share this little gift with my grandparents as they had always encouraged my singing. I enjoyed feeling the power of my voice and connecting with the spirit of Jewish music. It is like I connect with some deep, innermost place that aligns me with my ancestors. I forgot some of the words and made them up as I sang, but in that crowd, no one knew. That was a small triumph for me. I could feel the love and support from the audience, especially my grandparents. They were so proud that I sang well and that I know Hebrew prayers as they weren't very religious so they valued my knowledge and education immensely.

After graduating from college, Ron and I took a two-month trip to Greece and Israel to decide where to move. The idea had surfaced late one night after watching the movie, "Shirley Valentine," in which an unfulfilled British housewife moves to Greece on a whim. We were so touched by it that when it ended, we ran out to sit by the pool to discuss how we could make our lives more meaningful. We both sensed that we needed to be courageous in order to take advantage of this special time in our lives. We also knew that we had to decide where to live: San Diego where my parents had recently moved or Israel to join Ron's family.

We had the most amazing adventures in Greece. We even went to Mykonos and found the exact location where "Shirley Valentine" had been filmed. We explored our living options and even entertained the idea of moving to Greece where, hypothetically, Ron could make a living renting out windsurfing equipment to tourists. Despite the beautiful surroundings, I had a difficult time relaxing while considering our possibilities. I was in a panic, and it kept me from fully enjoying the trip.

Ultimately, we decided to move to San Diego to be closer to my parents. Even though I felt like my parents had abandoned me with every move they made, I didn't want to abandon them. The fact that my parents had been laying a ton of guilt on me to move there may have played a role in my decision, but it did seem natural for us to stay together. And San Diego is a beautiful place, so that was attractive as well.

After working at Blockbuster Video for a week, I got my first "real" job with a boutique recruiting-and-consulting firm. This was a wonderful first job. Not only was I using "behavioral interviewing" (a technique that asks open-ended questions about past work experiences), but I was also training clients on how to use the recruiting techniques internally; I was involved with selling and marketing, and coaching others on how to be better leaders. Not bad for a first job out of college. The job turned out to be really meaningful for me because I was doing work that connected with my passion to help people live meaningful lives. I felt important to be interacting with senior-level leaders and powerful to be impacting a candidate's chances of getting the job. It also offered growth opportunities, and validated the premise that I could make money doing something I enjoyed. I was kind of laughing in my parents' faces??

*See! What I love has value!*

Even though I wasn't making a tremendous amount of money, it was my first real paycheck and I felt rich.

During that time, I decided to sign up for a singing class at the community college. I hadn't been singing for quite a while (aside from perpetually singing in the shower and car). A part of me missed the creative environment, and I wanted to find a way to taste it ever so slightly.

Each week, we were assigned songs from various genres to perform for the class. Despite my being a nervous wreck, my voice was as strong as ever. But my fear had made me forget how to move my hands while singing and they were glued to my sides, completely numb and asleep. My perfectionism was definitely in the driver's seat. I was afraid that I would miss notes and that I wouldn't sound good. I was imagining that people were judging my voice and thinking,

*She sucks.*

Most of all, I was judging myself, thinking,

*Who do you think you are, singing in public?*
*You already tried that and failed — let it go!*
*You will never be a successful performer.*

My brain seemed to be taking over my heart and body saying,

*I am your master. You will only listen to me and therefore, you cannot move your body or feel your heart.*

It was so bad that I literally wrote a script outlining when to make certain hand movements to force myself to move my body, even slightly. I barely glanced at my hand-movement notes while practicing since; theoretically, I knew how I wanted to move. My challenge was to make the movement *while* singing. I became focused on memorizing the moves (again, addicted to the head) instead of letting my body and heart lead me.

Fear and embarrassment had never before gripped me so dramatically, but I still wanted to sing and feel the joy of the music. I knew my voice was sounding amazing but the rest of my body was frozen. It was like I wanted the feeling of singing in the shower while unknowingly entertaining an audience. I wanted people to hear me, but didn't want to feel obligated to entertain them or look them in the eye.

That was the first time I had sung, "I Dreamed a Dream" from "Les Miserables," a song filled with much personal meaning for me. I felt like I had lost my own life-long dream to sing. When I went to see the musical, I sat in my seat with tears streaming down my face for much of the production. I imagined myself performing in the play and being on the other side of the curtain wanting to peek out at the audience; I was preparing for my solo and feeling the audience taking in my songs.

During the song, "I Dreamed a Dream" my tears fell like rain. I knew that if it had been me up there singing that song with all my heart, I would have been able to truly move the audience. The truth of the matter was that I knew my dream was dead. I even imagined myself lying in a coffin as my family shoveled dirt on top of me: my creativity was being buried alive at the tender age of 25.

Not long after I had learned that song, I visited my mom's parents in Florida. They were miserable people and, by then, very old. They asked me to sing a song and "I Dreamed a Dream" seemed appropriate. I sang with all my heart thinking about their lives. I thought about how they had been so focused on being right that they had driven away all of those who had loved them. Singing it was a rebellious act, and I could feel my body shaking with emotion as I delivered the message.

My eyes welled up with tears, which made it difficult to continue singing the verse,

*"I had a dream my life would be so different from this hell
I'm living. So different now from what it seemed.
Now life has killed the dream I dreamed."*

When I finished, I sat silent for a moment before my grandfather said apathetically,

*"They don't write show tunes like they used to — there was nothing sing-able in that show."*

Obviously my message had been lost on him. I was shocked and saddened by his cold response.

The final song for my class was coming up, and I was determined to make myself move my hands during my performance. With much practice and effort, I made myself move my body very mechanically, but I was still avoiding eye contact with the audience. That was just too challenging for me. I was proud of myself that I stayed in the class and pushed myself. I was also completely frustrated and confused.

*Why did I have to keep pushing myself?*
*Why couldn't I be satisfied with singing in the shower or in my car?*
*What was wrong with me?*

One night, my parents had us over for dinner with some family friends, and a woman my dad had met at CinemaScoop, the video/yogurt store he had opened in San Diego. Her name was Kimberly and she was a singer, among other things. She professed to know every song ever written and boasted about having sung in front of thousands of people. At some point, my dad cut in to say,

*"Well, my daughter is a singer as well. She sang in front of five people in a bar."*

I don't know why he felt compelled to make such a statement. I think Kimberly may have been irritating him. Did he mean to embarrass me like that? Didn't he realize that it would make me feel like crap? What point was he trying to make? That I'm a pathetic loser? Was I an embarrassment to him because I wasn't as ridiculously boastful like Kimberly? I was hurt to the core. I couldn't muster up the courage to say anything because I felt so ashamed in the moment. He reaffirmed my belief that my dream to share my voice was truly dead and buried.

While I was in San Diego, I also signed up for an acting class. I was so excited while driving from work to the community college; it felt good to be doing something enjoyable for me. It was time to get back on the horse after my rejection from the American Academy. Who said I had to be performing for large audiences? Couldn't I just do this for me?

I enjoyed the classes even though I was still being overly critical of my own acting abilities. I was assigned a scene from the movie, "'Night Mother" in which the character shoots herself in the last scene. Since it was such a challenging role, I attempted to utilize the American Academy of Dramatic Arts method. I created a character biography, attaching real life moments to different beats in the scene. I still didn't feel like I knew what I was doing or that I was believable despite my best efforts. I was so inside my head. Trying to memorize the emotions of real-life events in order to draw upon them during a scene was just too complicated and cumbersome. I think it took me away from the scene.

But on some level, it must've worked in performance because I heard the gasp of the audience after pulling the trigger. I did receive compliments, but I wasn't very pleased or fulfilled by my acting performance. It just felt too difficult and belabored; it hadn't flowed. I just kept reminding myself that there was no way I was going to pull it off and be believable.

*Another dream down the drain,* I thought.

My dad's video/yogurt store went down the drain as well, and he was forced to declare bankruptcy. That was a shock for me since he had been a successful business person for his entire career. My parents had moved from their gorgeous condo across from the beach in Del Mar to a nice apartment in Solana Beach, and my dad was scrambling to pay off debts he owed to people. We bonded while trying to find a way to make it through.

Ron had been working for my dad so he now needed a new position. He got a job selling computer hardware, and was enjoying his new role. My brother was pretty involved with drugs at that time and was living with my parents. One time, while exploring the many messy piles in his room, I found some white powder that was used to cut cocaine. That's when it hit me: he was dealing. Not a happy finding.

I shared this disturbing news with my parents and this forced them to confront him. Unfortunately this did nothing to inspire him to clean up his act. It was scary to watch him self-destruct.

Then, my parents decided to move back to Los Angeles. They were abandoning us once again! We had moved to San Diego to be near them and now they were leaving again. Suddenly the seemingly endless moves I experienced as a child popped in my head. Ron and I were at a different kind of crossroads. We were debating as to whether to stay in San Diego, move to Los Angeles or go to his motherland, Israel. We wanted to feel like we were part of a family, and that we would be loved and cherished. We wanted to feel part of a community. We decided to move to Israel in the hope of finding that sense of belonging we had both been searching for. *But would Israel feel like my motherland?*

My family was devastated by the news that we were moving to Israel, which was funny since they had they planted the love of Israel in my heart at a very young age. I attended Jewish day school from kindergarten through middle school; and my mom's parents were big contributors to Israel's Technical College, Technion.

When my grandparents heard the news, they asked my mom:

*"What did you do wrong as a parent to make Rachel move to Israel?"*

Unbelievable.

During the months prior to our departure, I was deep in thought. I had an idealized feeling that everything was going to work out well in Israel, and was excited about the adventure. I felt different, unique and brave as we shared the news of our upcoming journey with others. Our friends threw us a big going-away party and I suddenly felt a sense of belonging right as I was about to leave. Why couldn't I have felt it earlier?

I listened to the Natalie Merchant song, "These Are Days," and it made me cry. It went,

*"These are the days you might fill with laughter until you break. These days you might feel a shaft of light make its way across your face. And when you do, then you will know how it was meant to be. See the signs and know their meaning. It's true. Then you will know how it was meant to be. Hear the signs and know they're speaking to you, to you."*

I kept looking for *the signs* to figure out whether I was making a good decision; I was just following my heart and praying for the best. I was allowing my Performer's intuition to guide me.

I sat on our empty bedroom floor the night before we departed for Israel staring out the window towards the bright moon that illuminated our room. I prayed that everything would be alright. What was I getting myself into?

## Lessons Learned

My first few years after college were a time of great growth and adventure. I was thriving professionally and dying creatively. On the one hand I was letting my Performer take the lead guiding me towards where I wanted to live and what kind of work I wanted to do. I was gaining confidence as a working woman and was so gratified to be doing work that I loved and that made a difference. On the other hand, my Perfectionist was telling me that my dream to sing was dead and long gone. I felt so sad and hopeless as I let my Perfectionist take the driver's seat. Yet, somehow I managed to still move forward by taking singing and acting classes. I was feeling the fear and doing it anyway. Unfortunately I couldn't appreciate that about myself at that time.

**Deepen Your Learning**

1. How do you know when your Perfectionist is in the driver's seat? What thoughts and feelings do you experience? How does this impact your decisions and actions?

   _____
   _____
   _____
   _____
   _____

2. What scares you? Where do you feel the fear in your body?

   _____
   _____
   _____
   _____
   _____

3. Think back to a time when you felt the fear and moved forward despite the fear. What allowed you to take action in the face of fear? What was the impact of this experience? How can you use this experience to assist you in the future?

   _____
   _____
   _____
   _____
   _____

4. What was your early vision for your life as an adult? Where did you see yourself living, what kind of work would you be doing, etc.? How is your current reality similar or different than your early vision?

   _____
   _____
   _____
   _____
   _____

5. How much of the reality you have created for yourself is a result of following your intuition versus letting your fears run you? How could you trust your intuition even more and allow this to guide you as you continue to create your reality?

   _____
   _____
   _____
   _____
   _____

# 6
## This Land is Your Land, This Land is My Land??

Living in Israel provided many "opportunities for growth." In other words, I was triggered on many levels. I continue to learn lessons from that experience to this day. I should have known I was in for a wild ride by the way I was greeted by the immigration officials immediately after departing the plane upon my arrival to the Holy land.

They started the new citizen process by creating my Israeli identification card. This identification is very important as it showed my legal status as a new immigrant which entitled me to obtain certain benefits and discounts. After arguing with the clerk about what Hebrew name I wanted to appear on the card (my Hebrew name is not the typical direct translation. It is actually translated to the ancient biblical name of Rebecca. This is not a nice sounding name to my ear and I didn't want people to call me Rebecca so I asked him to stick with the English pronunciation of Rachel.), he asked me for my profession. I told him in Hebrew "Human Resources." I then saw him writing in Hebrew:

*"Secretary"*

This really hurt my ego. I stopped him and demanded that he change my profession to what I requested. He finally made the change after much going back and forth. I was in Israel for 15 minutes and was already agitated and fighting to defend my identity!

After being in Israel a few months, we built a small, one-bedroom apartment within Ron's parents' house, which I called "The Commune." I was touched at Ron's parents' openness in dividing their home and helping us pay for the construction as well. In fact some other brothers assisted us financially too. Behind our newly created duplex was a preschool with about 60 children, a small house where Ron's brother Gil lived with his wife, and a couple of acres of orchards. Let's say there wasn't much privacy for this American princess.

Ron is one of four brothers, and his family is wonderful and extremely close. They are all very nice and spend a lot of time together, but the whole situation was too enmeshed for me. In other words we were too close for comfort. Keep in mind that we had been married for seven years when suddenly, we were sleeping in a room that had an adjoining door to their kitchen through our closet. People often popped in unexpectedly through the closet (just like on the '60s TV show, "Green Acres"!). Admittedly that back door was convenient for me since it literally opened to the refrigerator and was close to the washing machine.

The family spent almost every Friday night together, in addition to holidays and social occasions. But despite so much togetherness, each time they would meet, they would kiss and greet each other like they hadn't seen one another in years. My father-in-law would get insulted if I didn't kiss him on both cheeks every time I saw him. That irritated me despite his good intentions. Why did I have to kiss him when I had just seen him five minutes before?? Give me a break!

I would sneak out the door on my way to work in the morning and look both ways to make sure there was no one in sight that I had to kiss. Then I would jump into my car and race to work. Success!! A kiss-free morning!

In an effort to break away and explore my singing in Israel, I met with an Israeli songwriter/musician and sang for him in both English and Hebrew. He told me that I needed to work on my pronunciation of some Hebrew letters. In my usual way, I took it as a rejection and quickly abandoned the idea of singing in Israel. I decided that I would be viewed as an outsider and, honestly, I was scared shitless to put myself out there to audition, etc. To tell you the truth, I didn't have any vision of what I wanted to do with my singing. I didn't know if I wanted to sing in nightclubs, perform in plays, or what. Since I was afraid of failing, it was easier to never begin.

Finding my place while living in Israel proved difficult. I held a few boring clerical jobs, which were hard on my ego considering I had been training and coaching executives at my last job in San Diego. Now I was making coffee for my manager every day – yuck! But I wasn't ready to change my priorities by becoming a mother just yet.

I was also frustrated by the constant spontaneity of Ron's family. The Israeli culture in general tends to be very spontaneous — they "live for the moment," which is wonderful, in some situations. I could appreciate their need to live that way since Israel is a country that experiences ongoing war. They never know if today might be their last day so many people "live for now" and don't get bogged down by too many plans. But on a practical level, it made it close to impossible to schedule plans with friends or family; I felt like I had lost most of my freedom and control.

I found out about an English-speaking theater group in Tel Aviv through someone I met in Ulpan, my Hebrew-speaking class. They were holding auditions for an upcoming musical-theater play. Despite my fear, I went and was surprised to find a lot of people in line waiting to try out for it. I probably hadn't auditioned in more than 10 years so I really felt like a fish out of water. I anxiously waited for my turn to perform for the music director. Then he handed me something to read; I can't remember what I read but I know it wasn't my finest hour. I was so nervous. Usually, I overact in situations like that; I try too hard and it isn't believable. I also had to sing "Happy Birthday." I wanted to sing something else but it wasn't allowed. I finally had a chance to show off my talent but wasn't able to shine.

I later found out that I hadn't gotten a part. Ron wanted to work on the production backstage, so I decided to join him. I had never done it before and it turned out to be fun even though I was bummed that I wasn't performing. I was so close to the action and yet so far away. I wanted to be singing and found myself judging the way the performers were acting or singing; I was thinking to myself that I could be doing a better job.

Despite my discomfort, I started to make nice acquaintances. It was comforting to be around other English-speaking people. My Perfectionist convinced me that I was expected to speak, read, and write Hebrew like a native. The truth was that I was quite proficient in Hebrew but would often wind up laughing five minutes after everyone else got the joke. I felt like an idiot if I started to suddenly laugh a little too late, or exclaim,

*"I got it!"*

If I needed to ask my husband for a translation of some slang expression, then he found it difficult to be present in the conversation. I felt such pressure to fit in by speaking Hebrew. I didn't want to speak English; I wanted to fit in with the Israeli culture. Sometimes I wouldn't understand what people were saying but I was too embarrassed to ask so I would pretend like I understood and laugh or smile. I felt stupid, different and alone.

For the after-production party, Ron and I created a parody of one of the songs from the show. It was a great opportunity for me to show off my voice. Ron and I had fun creating the lyrics together and we sang a duet. It was the first time my peers were hearing me sing, and my whole body was shaking. We sang and I did a great imitation of the musical director. Everyone laughed, and I knew they were impressed with my singing.

Not long after that, the theater group was having a talent show. I prepared a monologue from Neil Simon's "The Good Doctor" that I had performed in high school. It was a scene set in Russia where the director sitting at the back of the theater asks a young girl questions during an audition while she is alone on stage. Ron played the director and, in reality, directed the scene, as well. We practiced and practiced before doing a dress rehearsal the night before the show, in front of another director. She tore me apart! She told me it wasn't believable and asked me to consider "other ways to play the character." Once again, a critique took me straight to my perfectionism.

I reviewed her feedback with Ron and, after tearing myself apart, decided to accept some of her suggestions while letting others go. I reminded myself that I was good and to not take everything she said to heart. The night of the performance I entered the stage, my heart pounding a million miles a minute (that actually fit the character since she was about to audition). Ron sat in the back of the theater and called out his lines. I felt connected to him and to the character. Just then, I heard laughter from the audience — a good sign! I became more comfortable, remembered all my lines and made it through.

Some of my Israeli family actually came to see the show. It was nice to have people there to support me in a foreign land. I felt like we did a decent job but, of course, I would only accept that assessment if outsiders confirmed it. Always in need of the external validation! My family did say that they enjoyed the evening and my performance. Could I believe them or were they just being nice? (After all, I had gotten laughs from the audience.) I didn't know if I had incorporated all the changes the director had suggested, but I was proud of myself for getting out there and doing something instead of just standing on the sidelines or backstage.

Well, I must've done something right because not long after that, the musical director told me he was considering me for the lead role in a new musical. I couldn't believe it! Finally, I would have my opportunity to shine. Finally someone, other than my friends and relatives, was acknowledging my talent. I knew I had achieved something by having been a member of the theater group and in the running for a lead role.

Unfortunately, that was around the time that Ron and I decided to move back to the States. Life in Israel over the soon to be two years had been incredibly frustrating for me; Ron said it had been challenging for him too, but now he claims that he had moved back to the States primarily for me (!).

We tried to communicate our frustrations to Ron's parents along the way. They usually responded in typical Israeli fashion saying,

*"Everything will work out."*

So, at some point, we stopped sharing and made the decision to return on our own. For me, the final straw was when my mom's father died. You might recall, Grandpa Irving was the one that scared me so much that I erased four years of math studies. Although he had not been among the nicest of people, I suddenly felt how far away I was; I was sad that I couldn't attend his funeral.

My newly found theater friends threw a fondue farewell party for us. That was the most connected I felt during the nearly two years we had been there. They served cheese and chocolate fondue and there was definitely an open bar! The evening was bittersweet because although I enjoyed the evening I felt like I was discovering too late that I had friends. I felt very similarly while enjoying our farewell party in San Diego before departing for Israel.

For a moment, I felt like I had friends who cared about me, and who I could have fun with. Why hadn't these people stepped forward months ago when I was alone, in need of friends? As soon as they learn I am leaving, they befriend me! It was a very similar experience to the one I had had with Ron's family. They only reached out and took an interest over our frustrations living in Israel after we had told them we were so unhappy that we were leaving.

We had decided to fly initially to Florida to visit my dad's parents on our way home to California. But two days before our flight, I learned that my only remaining grandpa Sam died. I couldn't believe it!! I was so close to having another visit with him. I pleaded desperately with the airline to get me on an earlier flight so I could make the funeral. I didn't want to miss it; I felt so connected to him and to my grandma Ruth. My tears worked and I was allowed to fly back, by myself, just in time for the funeral.

I stayed an additional week for the Shiva (Jewish mourning ritual), and had some wonderful bonding time with my grandma and my dad. For a week, we sat in my grandma's apartment while friends and family brought food and prayed with us each evening. One night, I sang a Hebrew song in honor of my grandpa:

*"Oh Lord, my God, I pray that these things never end.*
*The sand and the sea,*
*The rush of the waters, the crash of the heavens,*
*the prayer of man."*

I felt like I was on an emotional crusade to share my feelings and grieve openly. My dad and I had wonderful talks and took long walks together. We visited with family we didn't see often. I slept in my grandma's bed where my grandpa used to sleep. She tickled me every night and that became our little ritual. Those were precious moments. After my dad had departed for home, I stayed a few extra days and enjoyed some quality time with my grandma. I was happy to be there to support her; we had always had an amazing connection. Everything felt like it was unfolding the way it was meant to be. The fact that everything felt like it was "on purpose" and had meaning led me to believe that I had made the right decision in coming home.

## Lessons Learned

I was challenged by living in Israel on many levels. My Perfectionist was definitely running the show. She placed insurmountable expectations around how I should behave, feel and express myself. She demanded that I "fit in" to this new culture quickly. It wasn't okay to be different, unique or ask for special accommodations. I also learned about and struggled with one of the primary differences between our cultures – spontaneity versus planning. Part of me longed for the freedom to be spontaneous. On the other hand planning was one of the few ways I could control my existence since I was often at the whim of Ron's family's schedule. I came to realize how much I valued my independence and I struggled setting boundaries to maintain time by myself and time to be alone with Ron. Ultimately the challenge became too great and I had to get back to the United States.

**Deepen Your Learning**

1. Do you prefer spontaneity or are you more of a planner? When do you prefer either approach?

   _____
   _____
   _____
   _____

2. Think of someone close to you. What is their preference for planning versus spontaneity? How does this dynamic impact your relationship with this person?

   _____
   _____
   _____
   _____

3. How important is being independent to you? Think back to a time you felt your independence was threatened? How did you feel? What action did you take? What was the result? What did you learn about yourself?

   _____
   _____
   _____
   _____

4. Think back to a time when you didn't feel that you "fit in" and weren't included. How did this impact your choices, actions, and behaviors? How did you exclude yourself?

　　_____
　　_____
　　_____
　　_____
　　_____

5. How open are you to developmental feedback? How do you process this kind of feedback? What strategies do you have to stay open and receive the "gift" of feedback?

　　_____
　　_____
　　_____
　　_____
　　_____

6. Describe a time when you felt "on purpose." How did you know? What were the signs? How did you feel and what actions did you take during this time?

　　_____
　　_____
　　_____
　　_____
　　_____

# 7
## I'm an Adult Now

Once back home in Los Angeles, I reached out to an old college professor who had taught my first Management Development class for his input on finding a job. As it happened, he was the Human Resources director at EMI Music Distribution.

He asked me,

*"Have you ever interviewed and recruited candidates before?"*

I replied:

*"I have interviewed about 200 people."*

And he said,

*"Come in for an interview tomorrow because I need a recruiter."*

The next thing I knew, I was a recruiter implementing a behavioral interview process similar to the work I had done in San Diego!

I reported to the Human Resources manager, a beautiful woman. Pretty quickly, I learned that she had lost the respect of many because she was scattered and unfocused. About three months after joining EMI Music Distribution, I was promoted to her former position, Human Resources manager. A dream come true?!

It was all very exciting – I had a corner office with a couch, a stereo, and a great view. I even got them to put in the tinted window I requested so I could have privacy when dealing with employee-relation issues (an additional reason for the tinted windows was so I could have some privacy and be able to shut the door on reality for little chunks of time — heaven!) I was working for a record company that boasted owning 10 major record labels including Capitol, EMI and Virgin Records. I attended lots of free concerts, and actually attended a meeting on the phase out of cassettes to CDs. Unbelievable!

The job itself was a bit overwhelming. Suddenly, as Human Resources manager, I was responsible for all related activities for hundreds of employees in four different locations in California, and I had little formal training other than my college degree. Very quickly, I hired a recruiter and delegated the less appealing tasks like benefits to other staff members. I worked hard to establish friendly relationships with my direct reports. It was a strange and wonderful opportunity to be able to delegate tasks. Now able to focus on creating training programs, and on coaching and developing leaders, I became certified to administer a personality-preferences assessment and started facilitating team building. I was dealing with employee-relation issues and conflicts (that was the part I hated the most). I was scared shitless that I would screw up someone's life or be sued. I was in turbo mode, learning as I was doing. It was sink or swim. My Performer was taking the lead most days while my Perfectionist was trying to convince me that I would screw up. This was emotionally draining.

During that time, I decided to begin earning my Master's degree. Another employee at EMI told me about a program she was taking at California State University, Northridge – Counseling for Business, Industry and Government. Without much investigation, I embarked on what turned out to be a 6.5-year journey. I didn't realize that my program required 60 credits, while most programs (including an MBA!) only required about 45 credits.

I never sang during my stint at EMI. As a matter of fact, I was petrified of singing while I was there. How could I possibly compete with professional singers and celebrities?! It was seventh heaven to be so close to the music; I could almost taste it. Constantly given free CDs, I attended free concerts, and sat in on meetings when employees listened to and assessed new music. I felt like I was so close, yet so far. I didn't let anyone know about my love for singing. I kept it hidden, a secret.

I also felt like I had this new professional, "Human Resources persona" I had to embody. I was the rule enforcer, the "model citizen." Boy, was my perfectionism in gear. I dressed professionally and put on makeup every day; I gave off the air of being all knowledgeable and powerful. And I worked hard to gain the acceptance of upper management — I was proving myself.

But I felt very isolated and lonely in that job. I wanted to bond with other employees and be part of the action but I couldn't do much of it because of my own high expectations, and because of my role. Once, I attended a party hosted by an employee. People were drinking a lot and some even smoked pot. I turned the other way and pretended not to see any of it. Deep down, I wanted to join them. No one knew about my wacky, rebellious, creative spirit; I had kept her buried for quite awhile.

At some point, I begrudgingly accepted that I would never sing or perform again. I kept crying when I attended plays or performances. I was so sad that part of my life was dead. I kept thinking about the line in "I Dreamed a Dream" from "Les Miserables":

*"Now life has killed the dream I dreamed."*

I would go to crowded places like airports and imagine that I was an undercover superhero. My voice was my secret hidden power. I knew that if I began singing, the whole room would quiet down and that I could touch people on an emotional level. But I was a *retired superhero*, unwilling and unable to share my gift. The fear was too great. What would happen if they didn't like or accept my talent. To me, such a failure would translate into my being a meaningless person. I was really stuck, longing to share my creative gifts and, at the same time, so afraid.

My life shifted dramatically when I gave birth to my beautiful daughter Talia. Her birth made me realize how much I valued flexibility and autonomy. I started working a little from home and couldn't believe how much I enjoyed this freedom while still being incredibly productive and focused.

And then, there was a major political *coup d'etat* at EMI: the British invaded our management team. Our president was replaced and then, my manager was let go since he was aligned with the old president. A new English Human Resources manager came into the picture. I didn't see her much since she spent most of her time at the corporate office in New York. This was fine by me as she was cold and didn't provide much support.

I had been working my ass off for months, filling my old boss's shoes and attempting to show my new manager how valuable I was to the department. But I had an uneasy sense that she was going to lay me off. One night, I actually smashed my car into a pole in the parking garage at my apartment because I was such a nervous wreck. I had a feeling that my days were numbered. The next day, she called me into her office and told me that she thought I was wonderful but that she needed someone with "a different skill set." I was shocked, but my Professional helped me act very nice and cordial in the moment. I was stunned that she didn't need me to stay and finish up any of my work — I could leave immediately! What a punch in my ego's stomach. I quickly tried to make HER feel at ease as I knew it was an awkward moment; I think I even hugged her as I left. I felt so incredibly uncomfortable yet I was too scared to show my anger in the moment. I needed to retreat and process that tragic scenario.

The minute I left her office, my anger started to build. I knew that it was complete bullshit! I had been laid off because I was seen as being connected to my somewhat-ineffective former professor/boss. Even still, it was an extremely painful experience. The loud Perfectionist voice in my head was telling me that I sucked and that was why I was being fired. I ran into my large, executive office, shut my beautifully frosted door and let my tears go. I was embarrassed. It was like the line in that old Bee Gee's song,

*"I started a joke, which started the whole world crying, but I didn't see that the joke was on me, oh no, joke was on me."*

Everyone in the room knew the joke except me.

After a day of reflection, I decided to ask for a meeting with the "British Wicked Witch of Human Resources" to negotiate for a better severance package, and for cash in lieu of outplacement services. I told her,

*"Your decision was quite unexpected and I am still unclear as to why you are letting me go. I worked very hard here."*

She replied,

*"I know you have been giving it your best. We are offering you outplacement to help you find a new role."*

I said:

*"I know what I need to do to find a new role. Money is very tight. I would like to receive a cash payment for the amount I would have received towards outplacement. That would be very helpful."*

She agreed without much fuss. She was probably shocked that I had the guts to negotiate with her. It was a difficult and painful conversation *and* I got what I had requested (a very good lesson in learning to "ask for what you want!"). This meeting was a triumph for my Performer!

Immediately after the meeting, I had to head out to participate in an experiential workshop with my organizational behavior class, and I was determined to perform. So I went from the harsh reality of the "Dysfunctional world of corporate Human Resources" to the idealistic theoretical class on "organizational behavior." Wow, the reality was so different from the theory.

My Perfectionist's goal had been to attend the workshop without sharing any painful emotions; I would just pretend like I didn't just go through the heart-wrenching meeting where I groveled for more money. At some point in the afternoon, we were asked to do some assignment that triggered me. I tried so hard to hold back the tears but I couldn't and I broke down. I kept reliving the experience I had just had at work. My classmates asked what was wrong and I shared my tale of woe. It was a painful experience, and I was embarrassed that I had cried. My friends were very supportive and understanding though, and that helped me make it through the seminar.

As I looked for my next job, I realized how much my identity had been tied to my working persona. I was uncomfortable about not having a job because being employed proved that I was worthy of existence. I felt like a failure in telling people I had been rejected from EMI and that I was no longer employed.

I decided that I wanted to specialize in training and development for my next role. Instead of writing people up for not following policies, I wanted to focus on helping people grow and develop. The challenge was to show my transferable skills since, technically, I was a Human Resources manager even though I had much experience designing and delivering training and some experience coaching leaders.

Eventually, I interviewed at Easton Sports Inc., a manufacturer of sporting goods equipment, with over 1,200 employees in the heart of Van Nuys, which is not the nicest of areas. I arrived early so I looked for a pay phone to return a call from a consulting company I was interested in working for. I found one in a small, rundown strip mall. A group of Latino men were hovered together outside the mall drinking beer and laughing. That was quite suspect since it was only ten o'clock in the morning. As I spoke on the phone, the group of men moved closer and closer. I felt my heart racing and clutched my purse while trying to sound civilized and professional on the phone. What the hell did these men want? Why were they moving towards me? At some point, one of the men began asking me something in Spanish and I screamed at the top of my lungs,

*"Leave me alone!"*

The group of men quickly scurried away. Then, in my most professional voice, I told the man I was talking to,

*"I think I will need to call you back."*

I ran to my car and headed toward my interview. What a great first impression of the neighborhood!

## Lessons Learned

Landing the job at EMI Music Distribution was a great lesson in the power of intention. As soon as I got clear on what type of role I wanted, I started taking action and immediately landed a golden opportunity. My first real job out of college was filled with lessons that could not be learned strictly by sitting in a classroom. This was another example of how my Performer kicks in when I am placed in "sink or swim" situations. Somehow I manage to not only swim, but to become an Olympic diver. Despite my Perfectionist's best attempts at destroying my self-esteem, I have an inner knowing that I am capable of succeeding. I also have the dedication and perseverance to take continued, focused action to do what it takes to be successful.

I leaped into my Master's program without much research. This was another example of following my intuition. Perhaps it also exhibits a sense of laziness. It was easier to jump into a program then to do a lot of research on what I wanted and explore which programs existed. This was a period in life when I really began to compartmentalize my many roles. My Professional was creating a work persona. My Perfectionist quickly aligned with this persona making me believe I am not worthy unless I am very busy and working HARD! I didn't feel comfortable sharing my creativity or letting people know that I took care of myself and my growing family.

Leaving EMI Music Distribution was initially a big blow to my ego. After some processing, I used this experience as an opportunity to realize that I did not wish to continue doing Human Resources generalist work and instead wanted to focus on training and development where I could help people grow and thrive. In retrospect I am grateful that I went through this experience. There is learning in everything!

**Deepen Your Learning**

1. **Do you believe in the power of intention? Think back to a time when you had a clear desire or vision for what you wanted. Did your vision manifest itself? If so, what beliefs and actions did you take to help make your dream come true?**

   _____
   _____
   _____
   _____

2. **Think of a time that you were placed in a "sink or swim" situation? What was your initial response? How did you handle the situation? Did you ultimately succeed or fail? What did you learn from the experience?**

   _____
   _____
   _____
   _____

3. Do you find yourself compartmentalizing your life roles? What roles do you find yourself playing? How does compartmentalizing affect you? How does it impact your energy level?

_____
_____
_____
_____

4. Do you have a work persona? How would you describe this persona? How are you different at home than at work?

_____
_____
_____
_____

5. How does your work persona serve you? How does your work persona hinder you?

_____
_____
_____
_____

# 8
## Take Me Out to the Ball Game

The interview with Easton Sports went extremely well, and shortly thereafter, I was hired as the manager of Training and Organization Development. Sounds impressive right?! Except that it was a nonexistent role and department. I was starting from ground zero, a situation similar to the one I had faced at EMI. And, in the same manner, I was thrown into the deep end of the pool to sink or swim. The good news was that any action I took could only improve things. The bar was low in other people's minds, but it was extremely high in mine. I had to shine so I could prove my own worthiness as a person.

After interviewing "key stakeholders" to learn about the company culture and to determine training and development needs (administrative assistants were particularly helpful), I decided to create a corporate university that I named, Easton Training Camp (it fit in with the sports theme). It was a time of huge creativity and long hours; I lived and breathed my job for a quite a while. I kept getting intuitive hits about my vision and how I wanted to manifest it. I took tremendous risks like speaking candidly with the executive team. I consolidated all my data from my needs-analysis interviews and surveys, and met with the president to present my recommendations. I had never done this type of work on such a large scale before, and I had to influence the president in order to move forward with my grand design. Young, good looking and a bit cocky, the president was intimidating. When we met in his office, I brought in a large water bottle. As he showed me that my water bottle was bigger than his, he said,

*"You win."*

We laughed. The meeting was successful and he signed off on my proposal.

So, I proceeded to design and build a curriculum for more than 400 employees in three states plus Mexico and Canada from the executive level down to the factory worker. I developed a training-advisory committee to get input and help champion the program. I designed kick-off meetings that the company president and vice presidents participated in complete with Easton Training Camp posters, and company mugs and pens as employee giveaways. By implementing a competency-based performance management system, the company's mission and values were aligned with each individual worker's job expectations. Oh yeah, and did mention that I even facilitated most of the workshops myself? I really gave it my all.

I was so invested in my vision that I didn't mind being completely consumed for a while. I felt great satisfaction when some of the participants told me they found the workshops meaningful. But I wanted *everyone* to like the workshops and me for that matter (that was my Perfectionist coming out!). I soon realized it just wasn't possible, and that the learners needed to take responsibility for their own experience. I felt like I was having some impact, but I was on a lonely, uphill battle. My perspective was quite different from anyone else's in the company. My goals were to engage and motivate people on a personal level so that they could be more effective at work and happier in their lives. Of course, I didn't tell people that my secret goal was all about the people, and not so much about improving the company's bottom line.

My manager Jamie was the best boss I've ever had. He encouraged my creativity and really empowered me to take the ball and run with it. He was a great sounding board, and provided me with all the resources I needed. He was also the first to be a big proponent of coaching, and we met regularly. What a breath of fresh air! Conversely, my manager at EMI would take calls during our meetings. It got so bad one time that I went back to my office during one of his many phone calls. He came into my office a while later and asked,

*"Where did you go?"*

I said,

*"I figured you would come get me when you were ready to talk."*

Yuck.

Working at Easton was an amazing experience for me. I learned about training and development, and became certified as an instructor with a well-known training company that I will call TND. It was so satisfying to see my vision come to fruition.

Later on during my tenure there, a colleague took me to a Mexican restaurant where patrons sang karaoke at lunchtime. After much hesitation, I eventually signed up to sing the only country song I knew, "Strawberry Wine." I heard it while at EMI and had been singing it secretly for years. It's a song about first love, and it sometimes made me cry because it brought back memories of the excitement and innocence of young love. Before my name was called, I got so nervous that I was running to the bathroom every five minutes, drinking hot water and lemon, and generally freaking out. For years, I had hidden the fact that I was a singer and, suddenly, for a brief moment, I let down my guard and was coming out of the closet.

Of course, the MC called my name during one of my countless trips to the bathroom. I ran out of the bathroom, grabbed the microphone and told the audience that I had never sung this song in public. My whole body was shaking, as the MC put on the song. I slowly started to focus on the touching music and began to breathe. I kept my eyes glued to the screen with the words (even though I pretty much knew them by heart) so I could avoid looking at the audience. Towards the middle of the song, there is a great part where I needed to hold a very long note. I held on to that puppy and really sang it with my heart, and the crowd started cheering. It was such an incredible feeling to release my voice and let it shine — and to feel the acceptance of the audience!

When I was finished, I quickly ran off the stage. I loved the applause but was too shy to truly take in their acknowledgement. Then, the MC said,

*"It doesn't sound like that was your first time singing that song."*

I exited the stage shaking so badly that I could barely hold a glass of water...but I did it! I had gotten back on the horse and had been successful. I went back to that place a few times with only a couple of colleagues since I wasn't ready to share my talent with too many people at work. I was still very shy. Once I share my voice with people, I become afraid they will ask me to sing at the drop of a hat, that I will feel obligated to do so, and that they won't like my singing. One of my co-workers who played the drums, conspired to hide in the audience when he heard from another co-worker I was planning on singing. At first I was annoyed that he surprised me but then I quickly felt happy to be witnessed especially since he really liked my voice. I had a renewed sense of confidence that my secret weapon had been restored thinking:

*I know I can still sing.*

At work, I was treating all my workshops like productions. I would script each show, add brainteasers and activities, and bring candy and prizes. The audience was definitely entertained. I made progress integrating my creativity into my work. My Performer was slowly coming back to life and I felt joyful and more alive.

But there were definite challenges at Easton. After all, it was a sporting goods company where the executive team was primarily made up of young, macho males who weren't invested in becoming better managers or better people (which was always my covert mission!). Of course, they thought I was there to "get butts in seats," and to show that the company was providing training to its employees. My secret mission was to challenge people on a personal level to be all they could be; to live a life with integrity and authenticity. As I write this now, it sounds like a pretty tall order. It was no wonder I felt like I was a lone warrior on an uphill battle.

I was also part of an old-fashioned Human Resources department, and they didn't understand my role or why I was being treated differently than they were. At some point, they complained to my manager about why I sometimes worked from home, and wondered why I wasn't sitting at my desk a lot. Jamie put it to me this way:

*"I understand why your schedule is more flexible but they don't. I think we need to hold a meeting where you can explain how much it takes to create a training workshop."*

*"Wonderful,"* I thought, feeling a bit betrayed at that moment.

Now, there would be a showdown against five other people who needed me to justify my existence. He literally called a meeting so I could explain that each class I taught required about 40 hours of preparation, and that it was easier for me to focus at home. I also needed space to create huge flip charts; I had to defend being different. It was uncomfortable and it reinforced my long-term desire to open my own business.

It was a familiar feeling to the one I had experienced at EMI Music. I desperately need flexibility and autonomy to create and execute to my standards. These are my core values and I needed to find a way to honor them. I didn't like the idea of needing to prove my limited "face time" (meaning time spent sitting at my desk). I felt like I was being spied on, and like I was a little kid who needed to show mommy and daddy how she had cleaned her room to prove she was a good girl.

What does it mean to be a "good girl" in the working world anyway? My conflict was that I wanted to be accepted by the team without being obligated to be a loyal member all the time. One of my primary challenges is that my "little girl" is still running the show a lot of the time; she desperately wants to fit in and be accepted by the world so she won't be abandoned emotionally and physically. I want to be a good team/department member but I also I want to know I have the freedom to create space for myself when needed, and that I don't always have to follow the crowd and do what I was told. The theme returns again in yet another area of my life.

Whenever I feel too much pressure to conform or like I have to count my hours and prove my "face time," my Rebel surfaces. I start looking for ways to work the system:

*How can I leave early today without anyone noticing? Maybe I can take a little extra lunch? I came in early today while no one was here, so they have no right to tell me I can't leave earlier than normal today.*

I start to play all kinds of mental games, which take a lot of energy and creates even more separation between the others and me.

I also have this old tape recording in my head of my parents calling me "selfish." Somehow, I need to prove the opposite. I think it's fascinating that I gravitated toward a service-oriented role when I have an internal Gremlin telling me how selfish I am. Part of me may have gravitated toward this field to prove my parents and my Gremlin wrong. But my inner little girl still wants to be able to give freely without any expectations attached.

At a minimum, I secretly want to be acknowledged for my efforts. If I don't get recognized, I start to feel resentful. I might continue to give, but I now I am calculating tit for tat. I start playing the martyr as in:

*Look how much I am doing for you.*
*What are you doing for me?*

It's not a friendly game.

I realized I had gone as far as I could at Easton. It was pretty amazing that I had influenced them to create a training camp and to really invest money and effort in developing their people. Yet, I had a sense that they wouldn't be open to adding much more to the program. I was tired of fighting an uphill battle as to why we needed to develop our employees to get bottom-line results. Of course, my real mission and passion was to help people on a personal level, but that was my little secret.

I started looking for other opportunities "on the down low." I was glad the IT department wasn't tracking my Internet usage because I was researching companies and opportunities during lunch, and making phone calls from the office. It was uncomfortable but I felt like I needed to get out so I had to do whatever it took. I also became very clear that once I finished my Master's degree, I would start my own consulting practice.

Ultimately, I wound up accepting a training position with Transamerica. I was nervous about telling Jamie since he had been so wonderful to work with, and I didn't want to let him down in any way. I didn't want him to think I hadn't appreciated all of his support. I didn't want him to wonder,

*How did she manage to find a job while she was working here? She must have been using company time for this.*

I realize now that my deep-down fear was that he would abandon me or turn on me. The truth was that my Perfectionist was the only one placing these judgments and expectations on myself. There is definitely a recurring theme here, don't you think?

Once I had spilled the beans and told him I would be leaving in three weeks, he was incredibly supportive and understanding. One of the things I loved about Easton is that they knew how to give a proper "goodbye" to employees. EMI escorted employees out with a security guard. But Easton had a way of letting employees leave with their integrity intact.

Jamie actually threw a going-away party for me at a restaurant. To my surprise, he had purchased a little plastic kids' tape recorder. He had also bought a karaoke cassette with songs from the '50s that definitely didn't match my voice. He had never heard me sing — but he had heard about it, and he wanted me to sing at the party. Embarrassed and uncomfortable, I felt such pressure to sing but I was too nervous. My Performer wanted to sing but I didn't feel prepared. How could I sing without having practiced beforehand? My Perfectionist did not like that idea at all.

At first, I laughed and said to the group:

*"Oh great. Maybe later."*

But then I was in complete turmoil, thinking:

*Would I sing?*
*They are expecting me to sing and I just want to drink margaritas, eat my food and have fun.*
*I'm too full and tipsy to sing.*
*What if they don't like how I sound?*
*The songs are all wrong for my voice.*

My mental list of excuses went on and on. I could feel the knot in my stomach growing.

*How can I exit gracefully?*

As the dinner came to a close, I said something lame like,

*"Sorry guys – I'm too full to sing."*

Eventually, they stopped pressuring me when they understood that I really wasn't going to sing. I was unable to sing that night; there was too much pressure, and the expectations were too high. My Perfectionist definitely won out that night.

So much for performing on demand. That was never my strong suit, and I am still working on it, but I have definitely become more comfortable with it now that I have embraced the fact that I am a Performer.

My first day at Transamerica was the most interesting first day I had ever I experienced in a new job. I walked into the huge building in Downtown Los Angeles. It was like a mini city complete with restaurants and shops. People were running here and there, and I felt lost trying to find the elevator and the correct floor. I finally found my floor and my new cubicle home. I hate cubicles, but at least mine had a window with a wonderful view of the city. That gave me some sense of freedom.

I was immediately brought into a training room for the new-employee orientation. I was excited about it since I would ultimately be participating in revamping the orientation; in fact, I would be the one facilitating these sessions. I enjoyed the orientation experience and was looking forward to my new job. Just after returning to my cubicle overlooking downtown (not a bad view if I had to work in a cubicle), I was asked to immediately return to the same training room for an "emergency Human Resources meeting." I was thinking:

*What could it be about?*
*What's happening?*

I was completely disoriented. It was there that they announced that there was going to be a reorganization of the department in the coming weeks. Excuse me?! Reorganization?? Oh my God!!! I was freaking out:

*What does that mean for me?*
*Today is literally my first day.*
*Will I still have a job?*

A million questions raced through my head and there was no way to get any answers. I ran back to my cubicle and could feel the tears coming on. I felt light headed. Thoughts and emotions were swirling in my head without any clarity. Petrified, I called Ron and tried to whisper while the waterworks were flowing; I could barely get the words out due to my shallow breathing. He told me,

*"Calm down. Everything will be fine."*

That is Ron's attitude towards most things. Sometimes I envy him. I was anything but calm.

It turns out that Transamerica had been purchased by another company the year before, and that this reorganization was part of the acquisition process. They told us that we would be receiving more information soon. I spoke to my manager who said that she had no idea it was going to happen.

Over the coming weeks, I learned that if I desired, there would be an opportunity for me to apply for a different role in the newly formed company. The head of Human Resources had been asked to leave and, ultimately, my manager decided to move to the South to take a new job. So there I was, without any support or direction, trying to contemplate my uncertain future. I did do a little work on revamping the new-hire orientation. Other than that, there was nothing to do.

I would arrive half heartedly each day uncertain of what the day would hold. That went on for about two months. At that point, I was about one month away from finishing my Master Program's Thesis Case Study project. I also learned that if I decided NOT to interview for a new role, I was entitled to an exit package of around $9,000!!! I wanted to bring in money for our family, but Ron was doing pretty well financially, and our expenses were still relatively low. Might there be some flexibility and time to allow me to create my consulting practice?

I decided to interview with the new Human Resources director. I told him I was unsure about my decision and that I wasn't certain that I wanted to interview for a new role. I had also heard that he wasn't that easy to work with (of course, I didn't share that with him). I had been observing the people around me, as well as the industry we were in. I have to tell you that I wasn't thrilled about working in financial services. Very dry and boring.

After much contemplation, I decided I would take the generous exit package and launch my own consulting practice. It had been my dream for years, and it seemed like God was handing me a present saying:

*Go fulfill your dream, whatever that dream really is.*

The vision wasn't completely clear to me *and yet* I had known for the longest time that I wanted to have my own practice. I had to be more in charge of my destiny to have the freedom and flexibility to be a mom, career woman, and a person who truly enjoys life. I honestly hadn't even contemplated the idea of being able to incorporate singing or performing into my life. That dream was still buried deep in the ground.

I made the best out of my four months there; I even finished my thesis project. I also had the luxury of sneaking out early. I loved driving to my friend Gio's house and hanging out before the kids came home. I felt like a teenager again, free and enjoying life. Here I was, 31 years old, leaving early, blasting tunes on my way to party with my friend. I wanted to leave my cares behind and escape for a little while.

## Lessons Learned

As I advanced into my career, my identity and definition of success became increasingly dependent on the external validation I was receiving from internal and external customers. My Perfectionist's priority was work and I did whatever it took to excel. I couldn't afford to fail as this meant I was also a disaster as a human being.

My Performer kicked into gear by providing me with enough trust to follow my instincts including creating a corporate university and following my dream to develop my own company. I recognized that I was extremely anxious and resistant as I embarked on any new project or change for that matter. Knowing there is a natural cycle to change helped me manage the process better. I learned that I needed to anticipate these emotions during change and know that eventually I will embrace the change and thrive again.

I realized that when I am totally engaged in work projects that align with my values, I am very willing to go above and beyond. As a matter of fact, I am enveloped by these projects and spend much mental and physical energy on them. If I continued to work at this intense pace, I also became resentful and then started tallying the hours I was putting in and comparing myself to others in my company to see if they were measuring up. It became clear that I needed to work in an autonomous environment where I had the freedom to create and follow my own schedule.

I discovered that I really enjoyed variety in my work and was excited to work on projects from conception through implementation. It was during this period that I also began to put my creative energy into my work. I relished viewing my projects as productions and was excited to make them entertaining and valuable for my audience.

I realized how much I truly am motivated by helping individuals within organizations become more self-sufficient and productive. I recognized that I wasn't really motivated by increasing the corporate bottom line. I struggled to find ways to convince corporate management that they would hit their numbers by engaging employees and treating them with respect.

The valuable awareness I gained while working in corporate America, helped me discover that I needed to create my own company where I had the freedom and autonomy to work on projects that bring me meaning and joy. I am grateful for all that I learned during this period.

**Deepen Your Learning**

1. **Think back to a time that you were engaged with your work. What actions and behaviors were you demonstrating? How many hours were you working? How did you feel during this period?**

_____
_____
_____
_____

2. Remember a time you took a risk at work? What were the circumstances? Did you jump right in or was it more of a calculated risk? How successful were you? What did you learn from the experience?

_____
_____
_____
_____
_____

3. Do you hold expectations to be acknowledged by others when you are giving or do you give more freely? What is the impact if you give with expectations?

_____
_____
_____
_____
_____

4. Are you ever conflicted with wanting to be included and part of a group while retaining your autonomy? How do you balance these seemingly conflicting desires?

_____
_____
_____
_____
_____

# 9
# I Did It My Way!

During my time at Transamerica, I started thinking about how to build my new business. In my quest to get some clients for my new business, I scheduled a meeting with the company that certified me as a training and development instructor (which I refer to as "TND"), and they contracted me to be a trainer for them! That meant I would go to various companies and facilitate their material without having to market my services and seek my own clients. What a relief for a new trainer. Plus, I really thought their materials were well constructed so I believed in the services I would be offering.

Jamie, my old manager at Easton, shared that they weren't going to re-hire my position, and was very excited about the idea of my facilitating workshops there as a consultant. So, I had two clients and I hadn't even officially opened my business!

I left Transamerica with much enthusiasm and fear about what the future might hold. I took a drive up Malibu Canyon and stopped on the side of the road, shaking. I stepped out of the car and looked over the side of a cliff. My heart was beating quickly. I felt like I was about to jump off the large cliff in front of me without a safety net. My Perfectionist and Performer were at odds. I was scared to death while knowing and trusting it was time to feel the fear and do it anyway. I knew that my Perfectionist needed to take a back seat and that I was delving into this new adventure no matter how scary.

It didn't take long for TND to start sending me to clients. I couldn't believe it but I was busy training with them pretty quickly. Then, I started training employees as a consultant for Easton. What an incredible feeling to come back there on my own terms, earning more money and continuing my relationship with them. As it turned out, my intuition about Easton was right on the money as they have yet to hire a replacement for my role to this day.

So I began the process of building my practice and figuring out what the hell I wanted to do. At that point, I wasn't feeling good about my work because I wasn't earning a lot of money. I noticed how connected my self-concept and happiness were to my career and salary level. So I decided to sign up for a second Insight workshop to assist with my uneasiness (Insight Seminars is a personal development non–profit organization based primarily on spiritual psychology, and Insight 2 is a four-day intensive experiential workshop).

I knew that I would need to surrender my ego (not an easy feat) and let go to get the maximum value from it; I also had a secret intention of being able to use what I learned in my coaching. I was prepared to take copious notes. It didn't take long for me to realize I was going to need to fully participate and forget about being a coach to get the most out of it.

There were about 80 participants from all walks of life. We met in a beautiful room with purple carpeting at the University of Santa Monica (USM). USM is an amazing school that specializes in spiritual psychology, and I plan to get another Master's degree there one day. I get so excited every time I enter that sacred building. As I walked into the room, I felt the warm embrace of loving energy. That space makes me feel grounded and connected and I can't help but be my authentic, loving self there.

Over the course of the workshop we spent a lot of time getting clearer on our Gremlins while identifying the qualities that we wanted to manifest in our lives. We participated in many processes to get clearer on both ends of the spectrum. During one session, I was instructed to visualize my Gremlin and really identify with how it looked and felt, and hear the message it was sending. As I struggled to picture its appearance, it knew that I was nervous about "failing" the exercise and bombarded me with negative messages such as:

*You suck*
*You are selfish*
*You are an imposter*
*You are full of shit*
*You are such a phony!*

Tears began to run down my cheeks as I connected with that old, familiar and uncomfortable voice within. At some point, we were asked to name it. The name, "Sally the Critical Stage Mother" popped into my head. I suddenly had a vision of my mom (even though her name is not Sally). I knew that Gremlin all too well.

I feel badly for my mom. She is a loving person who was brought up in a guilt-ridden and abusive environment, both verbally and sometimes physically. She wants to love and give but doesn't always know how. Her subconscious mode of operation is to judge, critique and find fault in much that I do and who I am. Her intentions are so good but her delivery sometimes pushes me away and triggers pain and insecurity. These internal seeds of doubt ultimately lead to my perfectionism.

Later on, we did another visualization or "journey" where we asked one of our inner guides to show up. My grandma Ruth was instantly standing in front of me. I was pleasantly surprised and so joyful as I looked at my loving grandma. At the time, she was still alive and living in Florida. She was one of the only people who had ever shown me the beauty of unconditional love. When I would visit her, she would always let me sleep with her and my grandpa in their bed. She would tickle me gently for hours until I fell asleep. She would let me eat whatever I wanted. She always encouraged me to sing and would sit focused, truly listening and enjoying it when I sang. She treated me with respect, listened to my questions, and shared her wisdom with me. Tears of joy rolled down my cheeks as I felt so blessed to have her as my guide on this important journey.

Our facilitator instructed us to follow our guide to three beautiful treasure chests. Each chest contained a quality that I needed in order to be happier and more fulfilled. When the visualization was complete, we were to create an affirmation around the qualities we saw on the journey. We were to treat each word as if it cost a million dollars. The affirmation was designed to help us be more of who we want to be by focusing on our essence instead of allowing our Gremlins in the driver's seat.

I struggled with that exercise. I would start to write, and suddenly Sally the Stage Mother surfaced and told me I was full of shit and could never have the qualities I desired. I began to panic fearing I wouldn't be able to complete the exercise. I started sweating as other participants were completing their affirmations and feeling joyful about their results. I felt my stomach churning and my thoughts racing, thinking:

*How am I going to complete the exercise properly and on time?*
*I don't believe what I am writing*
*I don't believe I exhibit any of the qualities I identified*
*I am so full of shit*
*How can I share this statement with others when I don't believe it myself?*

Sally was winning this battle until finally, I went with my gut and this is what surfaced:

*I am a trusting authentic woman, freely sharing my truth, peacefully giving and receiving love.*

I was excited about what had come out of my head and heart, and Sally immediately started telling me that that wasn't really who I was. Instead, I was a selfish, ugly person who was unable to give or experience love.

I could feel my inner conflict. The facilitator called each of us up to share our affirmations with the other participants and receive feedback on them. Nervously, still sweating, I went to the center of the room and read my affirmation.

When I finished reading, the facilitator unexpectedly handed me a mirror and asked me to look at myself. She asked me to repeat the affirmation and this time add the word "beautiful." I nearly died when she said that and started to cry. My stomach was clenched in a knot and I stopped breathing. I felt anything but beautiful. I was emotionally drained and had been going in and out of crying for hours. Now I was going to look myself in the eye feeling anything but attractive and tell myself that I am beautiful??

She told me that she saw beauty in me and wanted me to include it. How could she think I was beautiful?! I knew she was focusing on my inner beauty but it was so hard to buy any of it. I looked in the mirror and repeated the revised affirmation. I saw my red, teary face staring back at me. I could barely read as the tears streamed out of me. I so wanted to believe that I possess an inner and outer beauty, but my Gremlin was shouting so strongly to the contrary:

*You are ugly!*
*You are such a poser!*
*Your hair looks terrible!*

I didn't know who to believe. In the past, I would have believed the Gremlin without question. I had been told for so long that I was selfish that I just accepted it. Now, I was building a new muscle. I had more of a connection to an inner knowing, a voice perhaps greater than my Gremlin? I couldn't be sure.

I was also extremely aware of being witnessed by the other participants. I was a bit embarrassed and ashamed when my professional mask came tumbling down and everyone could see a sad, confused little girl.

The facilitator asked me about the Gremlin I had identified, and to tell her all about Sally the Stage Mother. She asked me to see her, sense her and to make her present. I could hear the old familiar voices conveying nasty messages; I could feel her power as she gazed upon me in total judgment. Sally was definitely in the house. Then she asked me to share my affirmation with my stage mother. I recited the affirmation again but I could still hear Sally's negative chatter (she wasn't buying it either). She asked me to deliver it to Sally again but with all my heart, as if my life depended on it. So I gathered up all my strength and screamed out my affirmation. To my surprise, Sally quieted down. She didn't protest; she listened and was okay with my message (for now, at least). But that was huge. Perhaps I was more powerful than Sally after all.

They instructed us to repeat our affirmation to ourselves 100 times a day for 30 days. The logic is that most of our subconscious thoughts are negative so we need to counterbalance them by bringing awareness to the divine qualities we want to manifest. Did you know that research says the average human being has about 60,000 thoughts a day, 95 percent of which are the same thoughts they had yesterday; and 80 percent of which are negative and subconscious? No wonder it is so hard to counteract our Gremlins!

At the workshop, we learned a technique of counting out 100 toothpicks to keep us on track. When I returned home, I stated my affirmation while sitting on the floor staring at myself in the mirror. Often, I would say all 100 at one time but sometimes I would divide them up. In addition to the required 100 repetitions, I found myself using my affirmation when I was feeling doubtful, on my way to a challenging meeting, or about to facilitate a workshop. It really helped ground me and reconnect me to who I am at my core. Of course, there were times when I was just going through the motions or my Gremlin would surface. But I was determined to keeping my commitment to myself and the Insight facilitator. The affirmation process was very moving and challenging.

I also learned a powerful concept for fighting my Gremlins when they surface – forgiveness. I recognized the only way to release judgment on myself and others, was to acknowledge my faulty thinking, release the judgment, and recognize the truth about the situation or the person. This is very challenging and powerful work.

The workshop culminated in our picking a project to perform as a way to exhibit what we had learned and what we planned to continue working on afterwards. I wanted to embrace my Performer by singing a song about love that a friend of mine had written. At first, the facilitators didn't like my idea because they thought it might not be challenging enough for me; that was really surprising.

*Who were they to not accept my project idea?*

I knew that my choice would be meaningful to me and it certainly would be a personal stretch. But I understood that they wanted me to receive the maximum value from the experience. I explained that I hadn't been singing in years and that I was very frightened by the prospect of singing. I told them that I would be singing from all my heart and would be moving and flowing as I sang. They accepted my idea and I began to learn the song and plan my approach to such a daunting exercise.

I set my intention to sing the song with all my heart by telling myself,

*I am owning my truth*

That was my mantra for the day. I picked the only "flow-y" dress I owned. It was a long, sleeveless, blue-flowered dress. I don't normally wear dresses as I don't particularly feel feminine and many don't fit me right. But that was the one long dress I owned that I felt comfortable in. I am a bit short in stature, so long dresses are usually out of the question but that dress turned gracefully when I moved. So, I felt pretty and graceful, and it called forth my soft, gentle strength.

The day of the class performance, my heart was pounding a million beats a minute. I was truly touched as I watched other members authentically share in their own unique and creative ways. It felt like an important "coming-out" party for all of us. Before I sang, I shared my affirmation out loud to help ground me. The music began and I found myself moving; I actually allowed my body to move as it wanted to while I sang. Feeling so connected and alive, I felt I was flowing like a graceful swan as I sang about the challenges of loving ourselves and others. At one point, I twirled in a circle with my arms outstretched. I was beautiful and free.

After I held the last note, I stood in silence with my arms outstretched. The applause was overwhelming and I forced myself to stop moving and make eye contact with everyone as I took it in. A wave of positive love and energy flowed through me. I had claimed my truth and now felt ready to own the fact that I am a singer and Performer. Later, I was sent a couple of pictures while I was performing: one of them was taken when my arms were outstretched and the other was when I was taking in the applause. Those photos are powerful reminders that help me re-connect to my most grounded and authentic self.

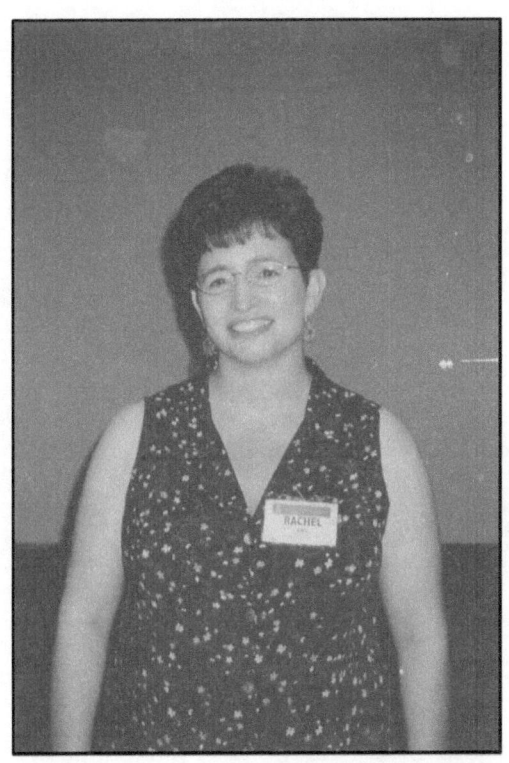
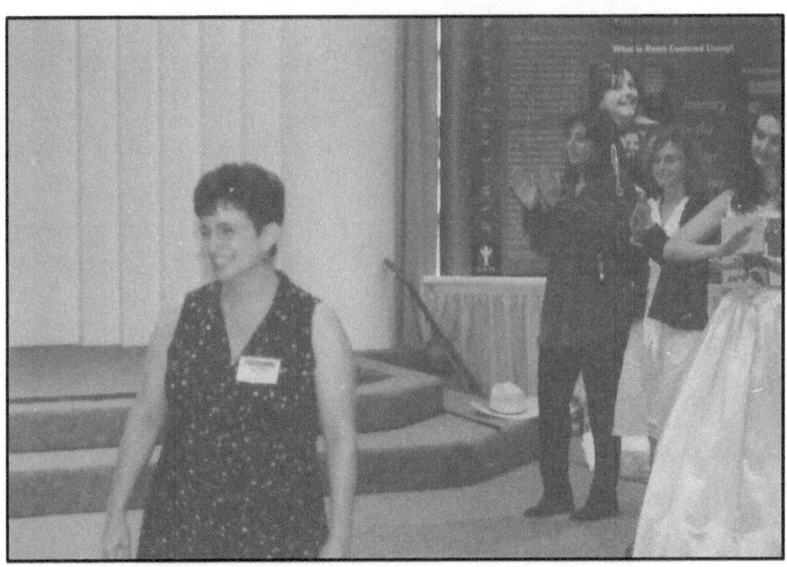

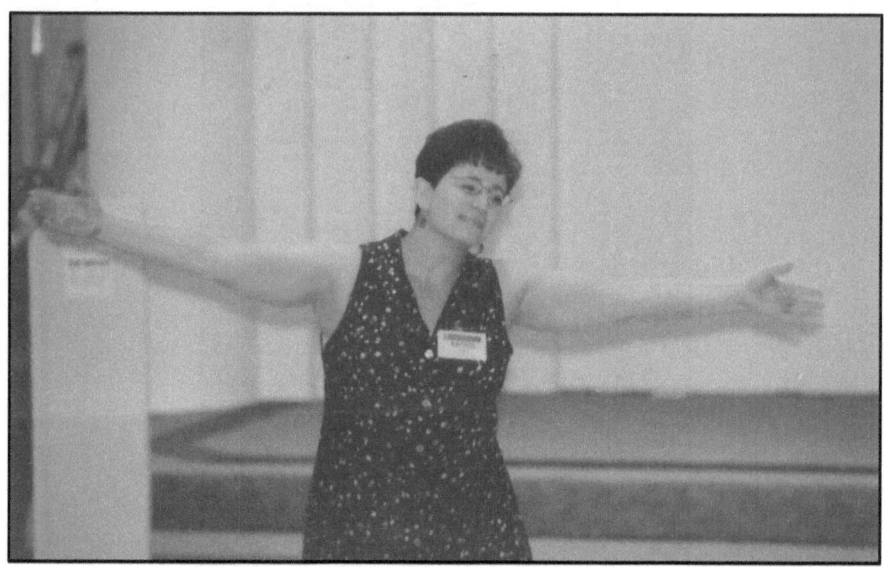

**Lessons Learned**

Creating my own business was the first real sense of freedom I felt as an adult working person. With this came much excitement and incredible fear and self-doubt.

I started realizing how much I defined success by my financial earnings. This was not serving me.

Having the courage to participate in self-development workshops was a huge gift to me. I learned about the crucial concepts of forgiveness and acceptance. I put these lessons and tools to work personally and with my clients.

**Deepen Your Learning**

1. How do you define success?

2. What messages do you tell yourself about how successful you are? Are these messages based on facts or on judgments about yourself? How might you shift these messages?

3. What positive qualities do you want to manifest in your life now? How can you manifest them?

# 10
## I Am Woman

Not too long after completing the workshop, I found out that I had become pregnant the day before the course had begun. One of Insight's ground rules forbids sexual relations during the workshop. I was using an ovulation kit so I knew that I was ovulating the day before the workshop when my husband and I had made love. How amazing to know that my son's first days had been filled with such incredible positive energy and that he had been a part of my performance!

After the workshop, I felt more at ease about sharing my gift. I wasn't singing regularly but I started to identify myself as a singer. I began integrating this wonderful creative part of myself into my being. It was a strange thing to suddenly self-identify as a singer. In the past, people would hear me sing and ask,

*"Are you a singer?"*

I used to grumble something like,

*"I've always had a passion for singing but I don't do it regularly."*

Now, I was saying,

*"Yes, I am a singer."* Period.

No excuses or stories or justifications.

Singing is a part of my inner being. Singing is the entrance to my soul. I am at my best when I am one with my voice. That is when I feel my deepest connection to who I am.

When I am "in the zone," I can feel myself breathing deeply and my belly expanding fully without any shame. I can feel the meditative vibrations of my voice against my heart and throughout my body. It feels like I am self-soothing with my voice. I can allow myself to relax so my body starts to move freely. No longer focused or anxious about how to move and when to move, I allow it to happen naturally and feel like a ballerina moving gracefully and freely.

When I am in this special space I feel things deeply and allow my emotions to come forward. Sometimes, when I am first learning a song, I cannot finish it without breaking into tears because I feel it so deeply. Granted, my perfectionism still gets in the way at times and I get extremely nervous and critical. But when I can let it go, I get glimpses of true inner contentment. I am grateful to be able to experience those brief moments of inner peace — and now I know they are possible.

The Insight workshop provided the opportunity to reclaim this special part of myself. I understood my Gremlins. I was also better able to acknowledge my strengths.

As for my business, it continued to grow. I was primarily facilitating workshops but I realized that doing training full time was exhausting for me. I treated each training program like a production complete with games, candy and brainteasers. I also became extremely tuned into the energy of the group and by the end of a workshop; I would be mentally and physically drained! Being on my feet all day was extremely painful and after a three-day training, I would be practically limping to my car. I couldn't wait to get home and put my feet up. I also had no patience to talk to anyone after facilitating; I had given it all away at the office. With no more empathy or patience to spare, I would sometimes get so frustrated and cranky that I could barely speak. My poor husband and kids.

Reflecting on my most gratifying work over the years, I realized I had a calling to become a coach. No, not a sports coach! A life, career and executive coach. I love helping people on an individual basis to empower them to maximize their potential and thrive, both personally and professionally.

I started taking coaching classes at a few different institutions. I made a conscious choice to begin coaching before completing any type of coaching program or getting any certification (otherwise, I felt like I would be listening to my Perfectionist Gremlin if I used the lack of a certificate as an excuse not to move forward). I had many years of Human Resources experience and a Master's degree in Counseling for Business. My God, there are totally untrained tarot card readers out there who claim to be great coaches, so why not me?? I think many women get caught in the trap of not moving forward with their dreams until they have the education or the document proving they are ready. Many men seem to just delve in without worrying about the formalities; they just trust that they will be successful. I decided to delve in like a man.

Learning and implementing new coaching processes was really enjoyable but, of course, my Perfectionist was still in there spewing self-hating comments such as,

*What the hell do you know?*
*How can you possibly help someone else when your life is messed up?*
*You don't know enough to help anyone.*

But that time, I decided to stand up to my Gremlins and move forward in spite of my fears. I acted "as if" I knew what I was doing. I was definitely afraid but I didn't let it paralyze me. I kept putting one foot in front of the other taking baby steps. I learned that the universe rewards action so I needed to keep inching forward.

I have now been in practice as a professional and personal development coach, facilitator and speaker for over twelve years. I truly enjoy the variety of coaching that I do and my work with groups; each requires very different energies and skill sets. It is such a joy to support people in getting clearer about their values and passions and then to help them move towards their desires. It is a great honor that people trust me enough to be truly vulnerable and to share their biggest dreams, challenges and fears with me.

I recently split with my business partner of five years, a major adjustment. Despite the challenges of divorcing, I am so happy to be on my own and be able to call the shots. My company is called RAE Development: RAE stands for Reflect, Act, Excel.

When I was creating my new website, www.raedevelopment.com, I realized that those three words perfectly capture my coaching and training process. I also recognized that my professional brand is all about inspiring reflection and results. I thought RAE captured this nicely; it also sounds like "Rachel" making it a double win.

One of the challenges of growing my business is that my true joy comes from working with the individual. Even though I have a corporate background and can "talk the talk" of the business world, I am not as passionate about it. I feel like I'm on a covert mission to help each employee personally and professionally versus being concerned with how to impact the organization's bottom line. That hinders my ability to pick strategic topics that companies want to spend money on, especially in a difficult economy.

Interestingly, I discovered that I thrive on coaching "Type A" personalities (like myself) because they tend to be successful "life learners" who are truly committed to enriching themselves and who are willing to take action. There is nothing more frustrating than working with people who say they want change but aren't willing to do anything about it. Perhaps that is my Perfectionist slave driver popping her head out. But sometimes, I need to remind myself that if all these clients had it together, they wouldn't need to work with me. That's job security, right?

Interestingly, I get consistent feedback from clients who tell me that I come across as someone who is accepting and non-judgmental. That is a learned skill in which I take great pride.

A key lesson I learned is that it is better for me to take some action than it is for me to do a "perfect job." In any case, people cannot relate to perfection; it's like holding up a mirror in which they cannot see themselves because they have become all too aware of their imperfections. In fact, I have learned that the more I share past mistakes and admit to my own challenges during a workshop or a coaching session, the more participants feel comfortable and become drawn into the process. When we admit our vulnerabilities, it draws people in. Being authentic and transparent is very powerful and it is something that is a part of my ongoing journey.

## Lessons Learned

After attending the Insight workshops, I started re-claiming my singing and self-expression as part of my identity. I reconnected to the joy and great purpose I found when I sang.

I was able to use the tools I learned to help me battle my Gremlins and reconnect to my true essence and the qualities I was focused on manifesting. I realized this was an ongoing journey and stopped expecting perfection in conquering my Gremlins once and for all. Our Gremlins are there for a reason. We are better off learning from them instead of denying their existence and trying to push them away.

I also became more in tune with what energizes and drains me in my work. I trusted my instincts and expanded my practice to include coaching. I further honored myself by splitting from my business partner and going solo again. These choices are empowering!

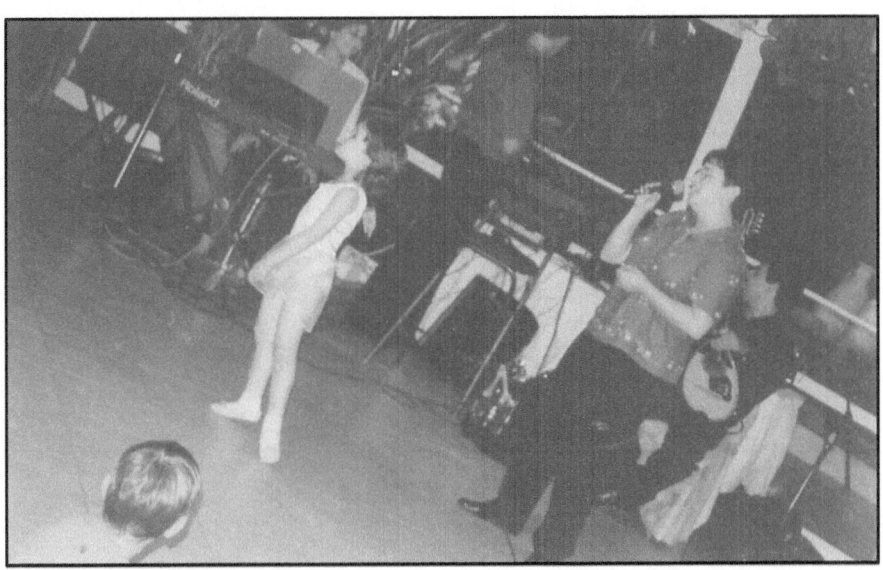

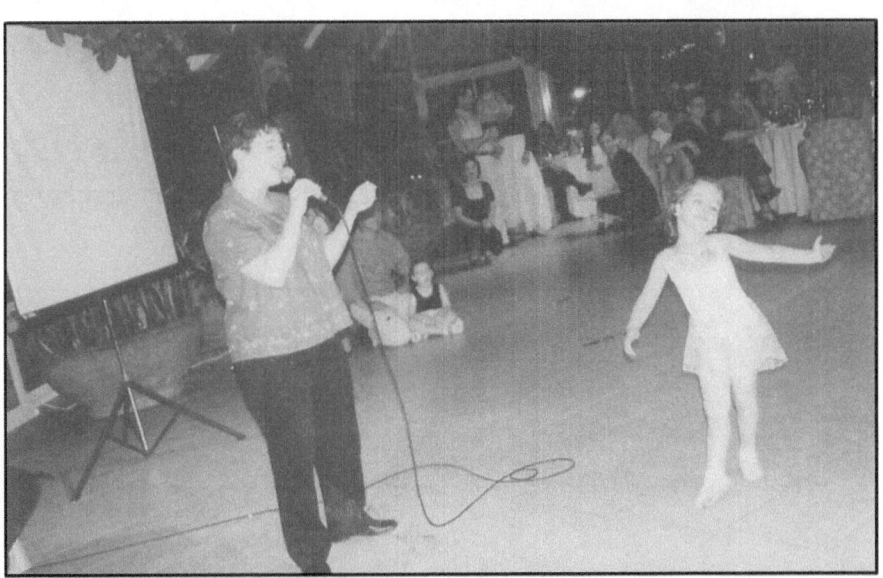

**Deepen Your Learning**

1. What brings you joy? When do you feel most free and alive?

   _____
   _____
   _____
   _____
   _____

2. What baby step action can you take by next week to bring you greater joy and freedom?

   _____
   _____
   _____
   _____
   _____

3. What aspects of your work energize you? What drains you? What can you do to focus more on what energizes you?

   _____
   _____
   _____
   _____
   _____

# 11
# The Accident That Was No Accident

One early morning, I was rushing to Long Beach to speak on the topic of work/life balance. My life in that moment was far from balanced. It seems like I (and many other teachers) speak on issues we are currently challenged with. It helps me stay honest, be vulnerable and walk the talk.

That morning was stressful. Freeway traffic was annoying as usual (one of the perks of living in Los Angeles), and I was very anxious that I wouldn't make it to my speaking engagement on time. I am a bit neurotic about being on time especially when I am the speaker who is supposed to have my life totally together (perfectionism rearing its ugly head). Stop and start, stop and start – that was the traffic pattern.

*Damn! I don't want to be late!*

Suddenly, a great Latin song came on the radio and I was totally getting into it. I was doing my best to distract myself from the possibility of being late. I blasted the music and — yeah! — traffic started to flow. I took this as an idealistic sign that everything was going to be all right, and that I would arrive in time. I started dancing with my upper body, singing out loud, and feeling the joyous musical vibe. I put my foot on the gas since traffic was now moving at a faster pace, and suddenly Bam-Kaboom! — traffic came to a screeching halt. I slammed on the brakes and barely managed to stop without hitting the car in front of me (thank God). Then, one second later ...CRUNCH!!! I had been rear-ended and then I crashed into the car in front of me. Not a pretty scene.

The first thing I noticed was that my lovely, hot Jasmine pearl tea had flown out of the practically non-functional cup holder, and spilled on the floor and all around the car. Then I realized that the hot tea had scalded my legs, and it hurt!!

The front of my mini van looked like an accordion. I was in the fast lane and could see that I needed to somehow get over to the right shoulder. My heart was beating a million miles per hour. I put on the turn signal and put my foot on the gas before I noticed that my car was barely accelerating. I was inching forward when I saw smoke coming from my hood. I needed to get to the right shoulder without getting hit again. I was talking to myself out loud:

*"Stay calm, keep breathing; just try to get over to side of the road."*

As I was maneuvering to my right, fighting a life or death battle, I suddenly felt a quick, anxious pang in my stomach realizing I wouldn't make it to my speaking engagement. I told myself that I would deal with that in a moment. I must stay focused on my mission to survive.

Somehow, my car made it through traffic to the right shoulder without getting whacked again. What a miracle! I cannot remember exactly what happened after that. I spoke to the driver of the pickup truck I had hit, and then I spoke to the woman who had originally hit me. She admitted that she had been speaking on her cell phone and wasn't focused when she ran into me. Amazingly, a police car showed up out of nowhere and ordered a tow truck.

In the midst of the chaos, I managed to call the meeting coordinator and tell her we had to reschedule. With the loud traffic in the background, it was all I could do to keep a professional demeanor while calmly saying,

*"I was just in a bad car accident. But don't worry; I am alright. Unfortunately, my car is pretty banged up so I will not be able to make it this morning. I am really sorry."*

She told me not to worry and to take care of myself before asking,

*"Do you want to reschedule?"*

Wow, I felt so much better since she was so nice and understanding.

*"Sure!"*

I answered with false enthusiasm.

*"I'll send you an email to reschedule."*

Click. Well, that task was off my list.

As soon as the cops left and I was waiting for the tow truck, a million thoughts flooded my head. I went into task mode; making sure I was clear on what I needed to do.

*I took the other drivers' information. I need to call my insurance company.*

Then, I suddenly noticed that my neck was throbbing. My guilty demonic side appeared thinking,

*Hmm. Maybe I can take advantage of this situation and get some physical therapy or at least a massage...*

True, my neck and back had been bugging me for a while but I was definitely feeling tension and tightening in my neck now. Would I be a bad person to use this situation as an opportunity to help myself? I suddenly felt like some sort of criminal scheming a terrible plot. I tried to tell myself not to focus on that right now.

I called Ron and broke into tears. My whole body was shaking and I was so upset, I could barely speak. I told him what had happened and asked him what he thought about telling the insurance company that I was in pain. He said,

*"Sure, why not tell them."*

So after our call, still waiting for the tow truck, I called the insurance company and told them about the accident. I made sure to mention that my neck was hurting. I was planting a seed I would harvest later.

That fateful morning of the accident was the beginning of an important life journey for me. I soon hired my friend Dawn as my personal injury attorney (you see, Dawn, I am finally acknowledging you). At first, I was hesitant about bringing an attorney into the situation. Again, I felt guilty, like I was milking the system somehow. After reflection and discussion with Dawn and others, I figured I had nothing to lose by asking for what I wanted, and trying to get some physical therapy.

Dawn recommended that I see an orthopedist who in turn, sent me to a physical therapist. Jim, the physical therapist, told me my muscles were extremely tight and that I need to start stretching day and night. It was here that I discovered my *psoas*. Who knew that this muscle could cause so much pain?!!!! I quickly learned the benefits of daily stretching. I couldn't believe that I was waking up early to do 15 minutes of stretching and doing them again at night. Some mornings, I was half asleep but I made myself do it. I became more flexible as time went on. That has made, and continues to make, such a difference for me. I used to visit the chiropractor regularly; I haven't made one visit since I started stretching daily! The physical therapy also kick-started my commitment to healthier eating and living.

But I digress. While at the physical therapist's office, I noticed a purple flyer (my favorite color) advertising a workshop – "Joy of Singing."

I was immediately intrigued. Joy of singing. Joy through singing. What a concept. That is exactly what I had been longing for over the past 20 years: a way to find joy while sharing my talent. I asked Jim about the flyer and he told me that Warren, its creator, was a patient of his. I made a copy of the flyer and immediately went into my scientific-research mode. While delving into the Internet, I learned that the workshop was about breaking through fear by using your voice and that the program had a new director, John Smith. I googled him and found out that he was a *trainer* with a large supermarket chain, in addition to being a musical theater director – wow! A coincidence? I think not!

Without need for any more investigation, I signed up for the workshop. I was receiving clear signs from the universe that I needed to take a leap of faith and take this workshop. How ironic that the workshop was called, "Joy of Singing" when that was what I had been seeking for so many years. I wanted to reconnect to the joy I experience with singing without obligations or judgments. But I had no idea what I could be getting into. I wondered,

> *Would this workshop take me in another direction?*
> *Would the experience have no impact on me?*
> *Would I learn that I suck at singing and that I should give up my longing to sing?*

I didn't have any of these answers. I only knew that I missed singing and expressing myself with my voice. I was excited that I wasn't overanalyzing it, and was following my instincts. My Performer was starting to have a voice.

A couple of hours before the first workshop, I stopped at a restaurant for dinner. While enjoying a wonderful meal, I set forth my intentions in a journal. Since I was nervous about the unknown, I had to use all my tactics to prepare for the special evening. The idea of being vulnerable by sharing my voice was another fear; it had been a long time since I had performed, and this is a very private part of me. But by the time I was ready to pay my bill and go, I felt like I had everything "under control." And then, I noticed that I had forgotten my wallet!

I couldn't believe it because I am usually incredibly organized. With visions of doing dishes all night in the kitchen, I panicked that I might miss my workshop. I asked the server,

*"Can I send you a check?"*

To my surprise, she said,

*"Sure."*

In the meantime, I called home to make sure my wallet was there and spoke to my then nine-year-old daughter Talia. She actually came up with the great idea to read my credit card number to the server and charge my card. Brilliant!! It was one of those "I could have had a V-8" moments.

## Lessons Learned

The car accident was a huge wake up call. My Perfectionist was trying to tell me I had everything under control by living "small" and in fear. That accident forced me to re-examine many important aspects of life including: 1) how out of balance my life was 2) how I was eating 3) how much and what type of exercise I was doing.

This greater awareness gave me the courage to reconnect with my performing via the Joy of Singing workshop. There are no coincidences. It is so important to be aware, pay attention, and look for the learning in every experience.

## Deepen Your Learning

1. **Describe a "wake-up call" you experienced. How did it impact your life?**

   _____
   _____
   _____
   _____

2. How effective are you at taking care of yourself emotionally, physically, mentally and spiritually? What can you do to nurture yourself more effectively in these areas?

_____
_____
_____
_____
_____

3. When was the last time you took a leap of faith? What was the result? What did you learn about yourself?

_____
_____
_____
_____
_____

# 12
## Please Don't Stop the Music

I left that restaurant feeling prepared to take on anything. If I could get out of that mess without a problem then, the workshop should be a cake walk.

The workshop kicked off with its director John belting out the song, "Joy." I was excited and a bit embarrassed for him — he had made himself so vulnerable by breaking into song without knowing us. I could tell it was a stretch for him, and that he was using his voice to model the challenge of being authentic and real for us. That immediately drew me to him and made me feel more at ease.

Not long into the workshop, we were asked to sing, "Somewhere Over the Rainbow," one by one. I listened to others sing while nervously anticipating my turn. I thought:

*That person really sucks.*
Or:
*This person is good — I bet I can't sing that well.*

When one woman was sounding great, I thought,

*Cool! Her voice just cracked.*

I went through a myriad of analyses and judgments while praying that I would measure up. I so wanted to be acknowledged for my talent — I wanted to "wow" people with my voice. But it had been so long since I had sung in public.

I finally got up to sing and I belted out the song. I could feel my body shaking, but it also felt so good to sing with the piano. I quickly felt comfortable and my voice flowed with the music. I had done it! I knew that not only had I "gotten through the song," but I had actually sounded great. It didn't take me long to begin to open up.

The structure of the workshop was that, in less than a week, we would meet three times and present a public performance with group songs and solos chosen by either Warren, the facilitator, or John the director. We participated in great exercises to help us move through our emotions, and to bond as a group. One exercise was to cup our hands in front of us and acknowledge our feelings before we sang. Most people then tossed the unwanted feeling away from them. For example, many would look at their cupped hands before singing, and say,

*"Hello fear,"*

before using their hands to throw the feeling away.

The next evening, Warren presented me with an incredibly challenging song, Sondheim's "Miller's Son." I couldn't believe he would pick something so difficult, and I was petrified. My Perfectionist was taunting me, saying,

*You can't pull this off in less than a week.*

But there was a part of me that was incredibly honored and affirmed that Warren and John had heard my talent, and thought I was up to the challenge. The song tells a story and is jam-packed with lyrics. If you are not familiar with Sondheim, he creates story songs with intricate melodies that aren't too easy to sing to. The character in the song is a promiscuous woman who shows off her sexuality and is pretty cunning. Wow! I had my work cut out for me. In addition to being challenging musically, the song exudes sexuality which is uncomfortable for me. I am generally pretty sexually shy so this was quite a stretch.

I attacked my goal of singing this song as I normally would: thoroughly. I set up an outside rehearsal with the pianist Tom R., with whom I immediately liked working. Not only because is he easy on the eyes, but because he treated me as a professional. I went to his apartment and I felt a little nervous, partially because of the daunting song, but also because he was very good looking. I got the impression that he was gay but still felt intimidated in the presence of such a handsome man. It was like being a teenager all over again. He helped me learn the song and challenged me to sing it properly. I loved singing with a wonderful pianist. As I became more comfortable, I could feel myself getting more into the music and getting out of my head. After our rehearsal, I spent every waking moment trying to learn the endless lyrics while driving. After much practice, the words and melody were starting to stick in my brain.

We were encouraged to invite as many people as we could to the performance. One of my biggest hang-ups was about inviting my parents. Part of the reason I stopped singing was that I felt pressured by them to sing on demand. My parents have a tendency to try to be in control of pretty much most things. I didn't want them to have any expectations or to pressure me in any way about my singing. I wanted this experience to be for me. I also was scared they would judge me for singing after all these years, thinking:

*Why start now?*
*Will this take away from the time and effort I put toward being a good mom and breadwinner?*

If I let them know I was in the workshop, I felt that I would have to defend and justify my reasons for deciding to sing again. On a deeper level I felt like I had to justify my right to happiness by doing something for me. I shared my concerns with our director John and he told me "when we have talent, we have a responsibility to share our gifts with others. I encourage you to get past the fear and invite several people, including your parents." I struggled with the concept of being obligated to share my gift but I finally invited them, along with some other friends. I figured it was polite to invite my parents, but then I needed to not focus on it anymore. I did my best to stick with that plan. I had plenty of other things to stress about.

I struggled to find something to wear. Since my car accident, I had lost some weight and was feeling better about how I looked. Yet, I didn't feel sexy and promiscuous like my song's character. I finally chose black dress pants and a pretty red shirt tied in the front over a nice black tank top. I felt pretty but was still wondering if I looked fat. So instead of focusing on being sexy in the song, I focused on being rebellious. Rebellion and the shock factor come quite naturally to me; I wanted to surprise the audience with my primal thoughts without being overtly sexy. That idea made me feel more at ease.

I had my usual jitters intensified 100 times on the day of the performance. I had brought my hot tea with honey and lemon, as well as my cough drops and water. I was continually drinking and sucking on cough drops. I had to pee every five minutes. While in the bathroom, I recited my affirmation. I recited my affirmation. I also imagined myself as a tree with my arms outstretched to represent my tender branches that were continuing to grow and stretch. My body was the trunk, grounded yet continually expanding and open. My feet were the exposed roots, just above the earth for everyone to see. I trusted that I was safe as I revealed my vulnerable roots, my soul. I so wanted to stay connected to this grounded trusting place. It can be hard to hold on to.

Moments before the performance, I was pacing outside the building reciting the lyrics. I was certain I would forget them. I attached certain body movements to difficult lyrics to help me memorize them. The technique helped me a great deal; it gave me things to do with my body without focusing on it so that my movements would seem fluid and natural.

It turned out my dad couldn't attend for some reason. I had very mixed feelings about it as he had always been a big supporter of my singing. But my mom was there; I had no idea how she would respond. We kicked off the performance with some group singing along with the audience. Our first song was, "Sing a Song." I remember feeling chills all over and thinking,

*This feels right and good.*

Finally, it was my turn to sing. I began by cupping my hands and acknowledging my feelings. I looked at my hands and said out loud,

*"Hello fear."*

But instead of tossing the feeling away like the other students had, I took my hands and laid them over my heart. I had the sense that I didn't want to get rid of my feelings, but rather work through them and embrace them into my being. My whole body was shaking and yet, there was a part of me that knew I was where I was meant to be, and that somehow I was claiming my truth.

I began singing and felt my whole body engage. I used the entire stage; moving, gesturing and singing that most difficult song. I embodied the spirit of its direct, confident character, but let go of the need to be sexy. Instead, I was a woman contemplating her options. She was calculating and manipulative; it just so happened she was talking about men and relationships. I felt like I was letting the audience in on how my dubious mind worked.

My movements were expressive, decisive and strong. I comfortably sang about my love options and how each of them, although attractive at first glance, led to a life I didn't want. The audience was laughing and enjoying themselves. I could feel myself breathing fully and feeling the warm vibration of my singing throughout my body. I love the feeling of the sound vibrating in my throat and over my heart.

Somehow, I sang without messing up the lyrics. My Perfectionist wasn't happy with the last note, though. Happily, I managed not to dwell on it too much. This was a sign that I was moving from perfection to being a recovering perfectionist. As I completed the song, I could feel the energy of the audience clapping enthusiastically. I forced myself to stand still and take it in. I wanted to acknowledge myself by feeling that loving energy coming my way. As I stood there, I saw my mom quickly stand up to give me a standing ovation — that still moves me even as I write about it now, six years later. My mom doesn't have the easiest time expressing her feelings; her standing up said it all. She stood a bit stiffly and uncomfortably as she gave an awkward, forced smile. I know she felt pride and love in her heart; it is just so hard for her to let it out.

That evening my mom my dear friend Gio and some other friends from the performance joined me for dinner at a Mexican restaurant next door. I so enjoyed eating and drinking a margarita. My mom told me,

*"You were great!"*

She said it with a reserved tone but I know she was glowing inside. She hung out with my friends and had a good time making small talk and letting them know she was hip and into the arts.

After the performance, I approached Warren and John and asked for some feedback and John said,

*"You really delivered the goods."*

Warren struggled to speak due to Parkinson's disease. He smiled and said "keep singing." People were approaching me from all directions to share their positive and enthusiastic praises. It was a real breakthrough evening for me on so many levels.

Now that I had finished the workshop, I had a renewed sense of purpose and knew that I wanted to sing and perform. I didn't know where all this would lead; I just had an inner knowing that I needed to follow my intuition without being tied to a specific outcome. I knew that I really did experience joy from singing with the group, and on my own, and that I wanted that heartfelt grounded feeling to continue. It was interesting how alive I became as I entered the Performer aspect of myself. I suddenly had this burst of positive energy; I felt proud and full of life. I had a smile plastered on my face the entire performance.

*I GET to perform.*

What a wonderful feeling. But my inner battle with my Perfectionist continued throughout the creative process. On the positive side, my Gremlin's fear of failure keeps me dedicated and diligent about learning the music and lyrics quickly. The problem is that the Gremlin doesn't want me to trust that I will remember the lyrics or to be grounded in that inner knowing that singing is who I am and that it makes me whole. I have continual doubts and judgments. The miracle occurs when I start to sing and I can let that Gremlin go. When I do, I open up my heart and can really begin to feel. Sometimes I fight my Gremlin while performing (I hate it when that happens). I am doing my best to be grounded and connected and then, I have a horrifying thought like,

*What is the next lyric?!*

At that point, I usually focus on a spotlight, if there is one, and close my eyes for a moment to reconnect. I hate when my brain fights me like that.

My survival instinct also kicks in. I take in and process data quickly in the moment; I don't stop if I make a mistake. I sense the need to pick up the pace or slow it down. I notice the audience without worrying about looking at everyone. It's as if, intuitively, I know what to do and who to be. I was born with this "knowing" and I just need to trust it and let it happen. That is what occurs when I am truly in the Performer zone.

Lee, a new friend who handled all the administrative issues at the Joy of Singing workshop, encouraged me to take some headshot photos. I also had a sense that I might be able to facilitate some Joy of Singing workshops myself, so I scheduled a meeting with Warren and John and they were excited by my interest. At that point, unfortunately, Warren had become very sick and John was working full time as a trainer for a supermarket chain. After our meeting, I had a hunch that I wouldn't be able to assist them much and wasn't sure if Joy of Singing would continue much longer. Sadly, my intuition was correct.

Soon thereafter, I heard that Joy of Singing was having a Master Workshop (that would be a Harold Arlen tribute), which would culminate in a performance at the Gardenia Lounge. I was so thrilled to be able to keep the momentum going with my singing, and that I would get to sing in a real nightclub. This time there would be group singing, and I would get two solos.

Warren picked a most unusual song for me, "Sleepin' Bee." It took me quite a while to really get a sense of this song; it wasn't quite flowing for me. It was frustrating since I had to perform in less than a week. My judgments were kicking in and I was wondering how I would pull it off. Warren kindly invited me to his apartment and began playing different versions of the song for me. Hearing others sing the song made all the difference in the world, and I finally found the groove. When I rehearsed the song before the performance, Lee, our assistant, told me that the song now sounded,

*"...like a prayer."*

I was deeply moved.

That time, I invited many people to attend including my grandma, and Jamie, my former manager at Easton Sports. That was very brave since up to that point, I hadn't let my corporate world know much about my singing (Remember - I wouldn't even sing for Jamie at my going-away party!).

But now, it was time to share my gift. It was a very special moment when I escorted my frail grandma to the bathroom and she confided,

*"I am so proud of you...you are living your dream."*

Those affirming words still mean the world to me. My grandma had just moved to Los Angeles from Florida, and she rarely had the chance to see me perform. And still, she was my biggest fan. She died less than a year later, and I savor her words to this day. Once again, my dad didn't attend; he was battling his own demons. I felt a loss not having him there.

That time, I performed with a spotlight on me for the first time. As I stood under the warm light, I felt it enveloping and protecting me, and I loved how I sounded with the microphone. I so enjoyed the group songs and loved feeling a part of a team. I was totally immersed in the music and it felt wonderful. In retrospect, I am so honored to have been a part of those musical journeys since that would be the last Joy of Singing workshop ever held.

**Lessons Learned**

Participating in Joy of Singing was a great example of feeling the fear and doing it any way. I faced huge insecurities and doubts and rose to the occasion. I forced myself to connect with my Performer and let her test out being in driver's seat.

This experience reconnected me to a deep place inside that brings fulfillment and is an avenue for me to authentically emote and connect to myself and others. I am so grateful that I created the opportunity to reconnect to this sacred space.

**Deepen Your Learning**

1. **Think back to a time when you did something just for you without seeking approval from others. What was it like?**

    _____
    _____
    _____
    _____

2. Reflect on a time that you felt the fear and did it anyway. What were you afraid of? How rational or irrational were the beliefs behind your fears? What did you learn about yourself from taking action despite your fears?

   _____
   _____
   _____
   _____
   _____

3. When do you feel most alive and connected? What can you be doing to manifest this experience more often?

   _____
   _____
   _____
   _____
   _____

# 13
## Defying Gravity

After the workshop, I decided to audition for community theater. I sat outside in my car before my first audition, shaking and barely able to breathe. I looked into my car mirror while repeating one of my affirmations:

*I am a beautiful, authentic woman, freely sharing my truth, peacefully receiving and giving love.*

My intention was to sing from my heart and to love myself for auditioning regardless of the outcome.

I waited outside in a little room filled with other actors and singers. Finally, it was my turn to sing the song I had chosen, which I recently learned during the Joy of Singing workshop, "Sleepin' Bee." Man, was I nervous. Unfortunately, I had the sheet music in the wrong key; the pianist wasn't thrilled but we somehow managed to improvise. Amazingly, they asked me to come back for a second audition – I was elated!!! How affirming. I ran to my car and began to cry. I had gotten a call back after my first audition! I felt like I was finally on the right track. Why had I waited all these years?

I became extremely nervous while preparing for the second audition, which would require me to both read and dance. What the hell should I wear? It took me a while to decide on black dance leggings, a sleeveless purple shirt and my dance shoes; I would add a black jacket over the shirt for the reading. The idea of acting and dancing were making me so nervous. I was having flashbacks of being at the

American Academy of Dramatic Arts when I had been hit with (by others and myself) so many criticisms including,

*You can't act.*

And

*You are a terrible dancer.*

The list went on and on.

When I arrived at the audition, I saw many younger people there waiting their turn. They were friendly and shared that they had performed in past productions at this theater. I immediately felt like I had no chance. I watched some of them dance as I waited; they were young and they could dance. What was I doing here? I was finally called in with a group of about 20 people. We learned two dance routines. I was so scared that I wouldn't remember the routines. I was working hard and starting to sweat. As I allowed myself to relax, I started to have fun with the routines and my face became very expressive. At least I looked like I was having fun even if I wasn't dancing well. They called us up in groups of three to do the routines; I actually felt like I did pretty well.

Now on to the readings: I was asked to read a scene with a male actor. I read it a few times, but I don't think it was my best work. It felt a bit forced and uncomfortable. It had been so long since I had done anything like that.

After waiting a couple of weeks, I called them only to learn that I hadn't gotten a part. I was disappointed and a bit relieved as I would have had to drive about an hour away for rehearsal two week nights and one weekend day each week.

I wound up going to one more audition for another show at the Odyssey Theater. I did a prepared monologue and sang a song. I felt very good about my audition and the casting person really liked my voice. After I left that audition, it suddenly hit me,

*How in the world was I going to handle rehearsals, work, and being a mom?*

I decided to stop auditioning and felt defeated. What was I going to do now? Was my dream of performing dead again?

Not long after my decision to stop auditioning, my daughter's school was holding their annual fundraiser and silent auction. I couldn't afford the $150 per person tickets, so I volunteered to work the silent auction and attend the cocktail party, which is the highlight of the night. I stood by an auction table for awhile assisting people, and then I was free to socialize and peruse the auction items.

I noticed there was an auction on two "vocal yoga sessions" with one of the moms from the school. "Vocal yoga" – what the hell is this?? My intuition told me to bid and, of course, I won!

It turned out that the mom providing the lessons was a professional opera singer who had developed a holistic approach to vocal training. I shared my DVD from my last Joy of Singing workshop with her so she could better understand my style and approach; she was shocked. She watched the DVD and exclaimed,

*"You are a singer!"*

She noticed the way I embraced the song, my phrasing and focus, how I used my body, and all of the emotions I was conveying. I shared my frustrations about the rehearsal schedule required for community theater, and then she asked,

*"Have you ever considered parlor singing?"*

I had no idea what she was talking about. She explained that I could either sing at a friend's house or rent a space. I could hire a piano player and charge the attendees. What a novel concept! My initial response was absolute terror. I also didn't feel comfortable charging people for my show. I processed this idea for a while, and then decided to move forward with a show but without charging people.

I contacted a dear family friend who has a beautiful home in West Hollywood and asked if I could hold a party at her home. To my surprise, she agreed. I then contacted the piano player I met at Joy of

Singing and his price was quite reasonable. Wow! It was actually coming together. I asked my friend Gio and John Scott to sing one song each, and had the piano player do one solo. A real show! I also asked John to direct me and, to my amazement, he agreed without charging me a cent. I felt so blessed.

It would be my "coming out" party. I invited everyone I could think of. My friends helped by providing food and dessert. I was shocked by how much support and encouragement I was getting. I was also a nervous wreck; my Gremlins were definitely at play.

*Who do you think you are?*
*You aren't so special or good.*
*What makes you think people want to hear you sing?*

Hello fear and judgment.

Moments before I entered the room by walking down the huge round stairwell to greet my audience (very dramatic), I could barely breathe.

When I got to the bottom of the stairs, I found a crowded room filled with my friends and family. There were 40 people there! As I sang a few songs, I felt myself begin to relax and suddenly felt as if I was singing in the shower, pouring out my heart and soul. In between songs, I shared my journey around my singing, perfectionism and fear. I felt so empowered and free after releasing the stories I had been holding onto for so long. My daughter sang a duet with me, and both my friends Gio and John sang. Gio and I also performed an interpretive dance – I was so vulnerable and brave.

The evening was a huge success! I base my assessment not only on the feedback but mostly because of how I felt: I had allowed myself to authentically connect to myself and the audience. It was an amazing feeling.

Not long after the show, I joined Cabaret West – an association for cabaret performers, and decided to go to a show at Vitello's Restaurant and Lounge to watch a member perform. It suddenly hit me that I could do a show in that venue. I also realized that my in-laws would soon be visiting from Israel and that I could surprise them by doing a show. That was especially appealing as my mother-in-law had always encouraged my singing. I called Vitello's and to my surprise, they agreed to have me do a Sunday night show. I had to guarantee 50 people and at least $1500 in purchased food and drink. I was so excited and extremely nervous. What the hell had I gotten myself into?? I quickly began strategizing how to promote the show. I used my marketing skills and designed a postcard and started sending announcements to my network. This was a stretch for me being bold like this with friends and family. It also helped to integrate my many worlds as I began sharing with everyone and anyone that I met that I am singer who is doing a show.

John graciously offered to direct the show. I really wanted a sounding board. I agreed to his suggestion to create a theme for the show; the theme truly found me. My friend Gio invited me to go paragliding for her birthday. I am completely petrified of heights; my husband had gone paragliding years ago and I had absolutely no desire to try it. After much contemplation and Gio's persuasion (she is quite persuasive), I finally decided to go for it.

Each of us would be flying tandem with an instructor at Torrey Pines where you take off from a cliff above La Jolla Shores. We waited for about 2 hours and watched numerous people take off and land. I could feel my anxiety building. We were told to put on our gear. I could barely walk. I met my instructor and shared my fear of heights. He said "no problem." Then he said "run us off the cliff and I will take it from there. Excuse me!!! I was petrified and annoyed as moments before this, I saw Gio's instructor doing all the running while she just enjoyed the ride. I attempted to walk while being strapped in with a lot of equipment, and my instructor glued in behind me. I was barely able to move and was shaking like crazy. I felt like a baby trying to walk for the first time. I took a few steps and then fell flat on my face. Very graceful indeed! I stood up again. I began walking, then trotting and suddenly running. As I took my last step off the cliff I yelled at the top of my lungs,

"Shit!!!!!"

And then...pure exhilaration and beauty. The instructor took over at that point and I could feel the cool air around me and the gentleness of the ride as we floated effortlessly over the ocean and multimillion-dollar homes. It was truly a "joy ride" and to this day I am amazed that I had the courage to go through with this.

I felt so empowered from the experience. The very next day, I went to see the show, "Wicked" for the second time. Just before intermission, Elpheba flies through the air with her long witch costume singing, "Defying Gravity." As I sat there staring upward, tears burst from my eyes. Defying gravity...I had defied gravity just yesterday while paragliding. On a more symbolic level, I felt I was making choices in my life to defy gravity whether it had been my own fears, perceived obstacles, or others' judgments that had been holding me down. It was in that moment that I knew the theme for my next show – defying gravity.

I began selecting music for the show. I knew I had to sing "Defying Gravity" and chose it to be the last song before the encore. I decided to reach out to a new piano player I had met at the second Joy of Singing – Tom R. He agreed to work with me. I love the way I lose myself in the music when Tom plays. I close my eyes while I am singing and experience glimpses of how it feels to be completely connected to the music. If only I could experience it during the actual performance.

I decided to ask my friends Gio and John to sing a couple of songs, a duet and a trio. From a production standpoint, I thought the audience would enjoy more of a variety show. In my usual way, I underestimated the amount of work the show would take. It wasn't easy producing a show with 3 performers with different perspectives and visions. I certainly learned a lot about collaboration by creating shows.

That evening, we surprised my in-laws by telling them we would be seeing a show and that I would meet them at the club. Somehow, we pulled it off. I made my entrance from the back of room, and could barely walk I was so uneasy. I kicked off the show with a Barbra Streisand parody "As If We Never Said Goodbye" from "Sunset Blvd.," The parody expresses her feelings about reconnecting to singing again after a long break.

Every time I felt like I was going to blank out, I would focus and stare at the light.

*Thank God for the spotlight.*

After a couple of songs, my mother-in-law spontaneously took the stage and announced how happy she was that I was singing and that she could finally attend a show. I became more comfortable with each song and started sharing many aspects of my life including how I met Ron, falling in love with Ron, my fears about singing, longing for happiness, and not living up to my parents' expectations. I ended the show with my paragliding story followed by my singing "Defying Gravity" and showed the video of me jumping off the cliff.

People were in tears.

I just watched the show video to refresh my memory and now I am in tears. I cannot believe how incredibly vulnerable and connected I was to have produced and performed in that show. I had authentically shared my soul with the audience and the stakes were high. My parents, family and friends who had been part of my successes and struggles were in the room. I shared my stories honestly and tactfully. My goal had been to tell my joys, struggles, weaknesses and courage with others through song. My intention was to provide a space for others to reconnect with their hopes, dreams and fears, and to inspire others to go for what they want and realize they can come out on the other side. As I revisit the video I can see that I was successful in reaching those goals, and I long to create that experience again for myself and others. It was an incredibly moving evening!

I felt connected to the music and the audience at certain times during the show and loosened up as the evening progressed. This is the challenge when I perform. How do I feel comfortable enough to trust I will remember the lyrics, song order, be authentic, feel the music, and of course sound incredible? Not an easy feat.

After coming home from the show, everyone went to sleep except for me. I was so amped. I sat in the living room and watched the entire show on our tiny video recorder. I was actually quite pleased with what I saw and heard. That was huge progress for me: I didn't beat myself up by analyzing every less-than-perfect element. My Performer was starting to win the battle against my Perfectionist. A precious, small victory.

## Lessons Learned

The universe rewards action. My proactive steps were providing fruitful outcomes which let me know I was on the right track. It was a time to start trusting my gentle strength. Amazing how things come together when our vision is clear.

I faced fears that had plagued me for years and found that I soared despite the obstacles. I felt "on purpose" and in charge of my destiny. I was able to do this by staying in alignment with my intentions. I knew the experience I wanted to have with the show and I kept that as my primary focus. Every time my Gremlin showed up, I went back to my intentions. This takes concentrated effort AND it can be done successfully!

## Deepen Your Learning

1. **When was the last time you consciously owned your power and stayed grounded in your strength? Describe how you felt and the results you experienced.**

   _____
   _____
   _____
   _____
   _____

2. Do you believe in synchronicity? Describe a time that this happened and you knew this had to be more than a mere coincidence?

_____
_____
_____
_____
_____

3. Describe a time when you felt you "defied gravity."

_____
_____
_____
_____
_____

4. When was the last time you lovingly acknowledged yourself? Take a moment and do it now. How do you feel?

_____
_____
_____
_____
_____

# 14
## Breaking Through

Pretty quickly after my "Defying Gravity" show, I decided to do another one. Gio had been a part of all my shows up to that point and we came up with the idea of doing a show together. We called it, "The Rachel and Gio Show." We planned to create a variety act in which we would sing solos as well as duets. We decided to work with Tom R. again.

Oh the joys of collaboration. We definitely clashed during the creation of the show. We simply had different visions and approaches to creating the show. Gio was pretty clear on what she wanted and how she wanted it. I found myself struggling to ask for what I wanted and was challenged by being in partnership. There were certain decisions that I wanted to make based on my past experiences. I didn't always want to collaborate; sometimes I just wanted to do my own thing. The experience challenged our relationship for awhile which was hard for me because Gio is one of my dearest friends. It brought me back to the realization that I need to be very clear when I truly want a partnership, and also when I honestly want to do things on my own. I am still learning that lesson.

I have some sort of pre-conditioning telling me it is the nice thing, or the right thing, to be inclusive. The reality is that sometimes that works and sometimes, I need to step into my power and keep grounded in my vision and convictions. I continued to learn that I can ask for what I want without the fear of being abandoned if the other person disagrees. Being abandoned emotionally or physically is my default fear. It has impacted my decisions in the past. I am usually attempting to avoid confrontation with the other person so that they won't abandon me. Generally, the other person senses something is off, or that I'm not being authentic, and makes assumptions. I eventually wind up telling them what I was trying to avoid and it comes out awkwardly. Then, the other person becomes uncomfortable and reduces their trust in me because I wasn't upfront with them to begin with. It actually creates separation, which is exactly what I was trying avoid. I found myself falling into this trap with Gio during our show; it was a great lesson for me.

The other observation is that as much as I feared being abandoned, I witnessed that my knee jerk response was to run away and distance myself from Gio when we weren't on the same page instead of dealing with it head on. This is a pattern I noticed in other relationships as well.

The honeymoon phase of my "renaissance" had worn off. I chose songs that represented a full spectrum of emotions and issues such as challenges with self-acceptance, jealousy, perfectionism (of course), and love gone bad. Gio balanced those out with softer love songs and standards.

During that time, I started taking a vocal class with Karen M. I thought it would be helpful to get some coaching before my next show. Karen is a veteran singer and Tony Award winner who has performed on television numerous times. The format of her classes was that each of us would sing a song of our choosing and then hear her critique. This experience was both good and painful. She was brutally honest, which I appreciated. I also think she has "her way" of doing things and, at times, I felt forced to fit into her mold, which may or may not have been in alignment with my style. One example is she kept telling me to limit how much I move my head and body while singing. Of course, I am open to experimenting, but Karen doesn't realize that my movement is a huge accomplishment and growth for me. My arms were no longer paralyzed by my side. Ever since I sang at the last Insight workshop, I had been able to move and to feel the music in my body. At another class, Karen said that my face was very expressive but that the rest of my body was "dead."

I continue to learn how to use my body during singing. There is a primitive part of me from childhood that doesn't feel safe while moving my body. That stems from being molested by other children when I was around 10 years old (needless to say, that had a great impact on my life). To this day, I have this "fright or flight" response that if I just keep still and don't move, I will be safe. I even remember that when I was about ten, I came up with the notion that if I fell asleep with my legs crossed Indian style, I would be protected (a very uncomfortable sleeping position!). Yet I feel quite comfortable letting my voice boom and soar. It is the opening to my soul; I share my heart through my voice while the rest of my body remains in fear.

As time progresses, I feel more natural and comfortable moving my body while I sing. I don't want to thwart that movement even if it might be too much. I need to build the body-moving muscle and I know that with time I will find the right balance.

The bottom line was that although I appreciated the feedback, it triggered a lot of old insecurities and fears, which was not helping me to prepare for my show. I decided that if I needed coaching, I would go to a private vocal coach Gio had recommended. It turned out to be a more nurturing environment for me.

Happily, our show was quite successful — we even sold out on a Saturday night! Vitello's was very pleased. Our duets had been wonderful: my favorite was an amazing duet arrangement combining "Happy Days are Here Again" and "Come On Get Happy" that Barbra Streisand and Judy Garland had sung in the '60s. My daughter Talia and I sang a duet from "Wicked" called "Loathing." She was amazing and it fit the mother/daughter relationship so well. I had even arranged for several of Talia's friends to act as a choir during the song, "Unwritten." The audience was both surprised and moved.

My singing the Alanis Morrisette song, "Perfect" was truly a perfect choice for me. It's about how parents demand perfection from their children and verbally abuse them when they don't hit the mark. Singing it was a bold move on my part since my parents were in the audience. I had set up the song by sharing that I was a recovering Perfectionist and that my intention was to promote acceptance and excellence in my children. I shared that sometimes the old tapes keep playing. I really wanted to make the song about me and not my parents. After all, I had embraced their messages and it was now my job to figure out how to unravel the old thought patterns and make different choices. I remember going back and forth in rehearsals about how strongly to sing the song. During my last rehearsal with the pianist Tom R. before the show, he encouraged me not to hold back and let it rip. And that is exactly what I did. My rebellious side was actually excited to make the audience uncomfortable with the troubling lyrics such as,

> "Be a good girl.
> You gotta try a little harder.
> That wasn't good enough to make us proud."

I put my entire heart and soul in the song. I ended with the lyric,

> "We'll love you just the way you are, if you're perfect."

There was complete silence. The silence felt like it lasted for an eternity. I think people were shocked and were processing their feelings. That was exactly the impact I was going for.

During that period, I also started leading the Torah service off and on at my synagogue. I am usually quite nervous when leading any part of the service. It takes me back to being a teenager and feeling my whole body tremble. Sometimes I question whether I believe in God and ask myself if am being authentic. Sometimes, I feel inadequate because I don't understand everything I am reading and don't know all of the traditions. Other times, I get nervous about doing everything right and not wanting to look stupid. But when I put all of those feelings aside and allow myself to become centered while chanting prayers, something magical happens. There is an inexplicable connection I feel in my soul and spirit; I sense it and know the congregants experience it as well. I cannot deny that I have some deep connection to being Jewish that is in my blood and on a cellular level.

Many people have asked me if I wanted to become a Cantor. In fact, they have been asking me that since I was 12 years old. I could never become a Cantor for the reasons I listed above. I also don't want to be held up as a pillar of society. I have many flaws, imperfections and a strong, rebellious side. I don't want people to be looking at my actions and expecting me to behave a certain way. In short, I don't want to be put up on a pedestal.

Singing in synagogue also brings up the question of just how connected to a community I want to be. Part of me longs to be part of a group and feel accepted. But as soon as I begin to feel that connection, another part of me becomes fearful about being obligated to give my all to the group. I know it comes from my family's high expectations. I tell myself that I am not welcome into the system or into the fold unless I perpetually agree to do what is expected of me. For those reasons, I am very conscious of what I say "yes" or "no" to.

I also find myself constantly judging and justifying how much I give in certain relationships. Of course, I also make those same calculations about others who are in a relationship with me. I don't like that kind of "tit for tat" mentality, but it is hard to break free from it.

I felt many of those emotions during the lead up to my last show with Gio. I found myself competing and judging. Sometimes, I wanted connection and collaboration. Other times I wanted to be free to make my own choices and decisions. I found it hard to ask for what I wanted because subconsciously, I feared that I would be abandoned if I took a stand for what I want.

*Oy!!*

For those reasons, I waited a while before doing my next show. I was also focusing on bringing in income, which takes away from my time to create shows.

Around that time, Ron decided to buy a stone restoration franchise and quit his Information Technology sales job. He took an equity loan from our house to finance the business. I had a strong feeling that we would be okay until that money ran out but that then, we would be in trouble. Unfortunately, my intuition was spot on. I will return to this part of the story soon.

I had always wanted to record music since my teenage experience in the studio so I decided to create a demo CD in between shows. I had taken a singing workshop and learned about Geoffrey T., a songwriter who had a small studio in his home. He was recommended by another friend as well, so I called him and scheduled an appointment. I noticed his 1940s apartment building had very cool architecture. As I headed down the hall to his apartment, he popped his head out to greet me and led me inside. I was shocked to discover how tiny his single apartment was. I thought:

*Had I made a mistake in coming here?*
*Who was this guy and how could he possibly have a studio in such a cluttered space?*

It turned out that Geoffrey had wonderful recording equipment and we worked on a variety of songs and snippets of songs. I decided to categorize the songs into three genres:

1) *Pop*

2) *Show tunes*

3) *Standards*

My goal was to start performing at events so I chose songs that I thought would work well at parties.

I quickly learned that Geoffrey was a wonderful pop/jazz piano player but wasn't technically skilled enough to do musical-theater pieces. So I brought in tracks from working with Tom R. and he was able to tweak them to be even better than before. I loved recording that CD! Once I got over the newness of working with Geoffrey, I closed my eyes and let my voice and heart soar. I needed to sing directly into the microphone so I could just move my hands. I could feel the music flowing through me.

Some of the songs came easy like "My Funny Valentine," "Happy Days are Here Again," "Natural Woman" and "Crossword Puzzle." Others were more challenging. We worked endlessly on the Sara Bareilles song, "Vegas" but I didn't end up using it. I would still love to sing that song, though. I was also challenged with "I Feel the Earth Move" and the most difficult one for me was Donna Summer's "Last Dance."

Disco was definitely a stretch for me but I wanted an upbeat party song. I found a great karaoke track and went to a voice teacher to work on the song; she provided wonderful feedback and ideas. I then recorded a section of the song, and was so happy with how it turned out. Geoffrey was able to manipulate one of the last notes to make it sound like I held it forever. Oh, the wonders of recording!!

Talia helped me design a CD cover and Ron bought a special printer so we that would actually burn CDs with our own graphics. What a wonderful family project! I was so grateful to everyone for their help. I started sending out my CDs to everyone and anyone I could think of.

I also joined a booking website called Gigmasters. I posted my song list and headshots as well as some of the songs from the CD so that people could hear me. I started getting notices about potential gigs. Unfortunately, I learned that that website is only good if you play an instrument or are part of a band, so it hasn't worked for me. But it has been invaluable to have a place to refer people when I want them to hear me sing.

Finally, I decided to do another show but this time, I wanted it be "my show." I wanted to be free to make my song choices and to decide on pricing, dates, musicians, etc. As a creative way to "fill the house," I decided to have two other musicians participate by singing three solos, three trios, and a duet with me. I thought,

*This is such a simple format.*

Every singer rehearses on their own and each has a following so we will have no problem filling the house. Sounds great in theory, right??

Well, of course my simple model was not so simple. Firstly, I had chosen a new piano player – Kurt. He is a wonderful musician/arranger *and* a total perfectionist. Each arrangement he created for the duets and trios (which wound up being quartets because Talia sang backup) were so intricate that they were challenging for the other singers. I had not planned on incorporating Gio into the show but I wound up working with her and John again.

I told Gio about my vision to utilize other singers and she said it would be strange for her if I were to work with other singers and not her. I felt awkward and decided to involve her in the show even though that wasn't my original intention. Working with John proved to be challenging because he had an unexpected work commitment that took up much of his time and energy. I had also decided to incorporate David, a multi-instrumentalist who wasn't the easiest to work with. His style was completely different than Kurt's. A consummate musician, Kurt was all about being a professional. David liked to improvise and groove without much rehearsal. Kurt didn't have much respect for David, and David was intimidated by Kurt. It was yet another complication for me.

I titled the show, "Breaking Through" to suggest that I would soon be emerging from the many challenges in my life including much financial uncertainty. Somehow, I was stepping forward courageously and pursuing my dreams and passions despite those challenges. I wanted to convey to the audience the range of emotions I was experiencing, and for them to be inspired to "break through" their challenges. The song that really summed up the sentiment for the show was Jason Robert Brown's "I'm Not Afraid of Anything" which tells the story of a woman who appears to be fearless. She professes her love for any type of challenge; she is bold and strong. In the middle of the song, she blurts out unexpectedly,

*"And David loves me, he's afraid to tell me.*
*And David loves me, he's afraid to hold me.*
*He's afraid to trust me, and he'll always be.*
*He's afraid of me."*

That section shows her true vulnerability and reveals that her strength is a cover up for not letting people into her inner fear-filled world. Oh, how I resonate with that song. I appear so strong and brave to many, yet deep down I have moments of fear and insecurity. I am constantly standing up to my Gremlins and learning that being vulnerable and open is truly powerful. It is definitely a journey.

For each show, I had traditionally chosen a serenade for Ron. But at that time in my life, it was challenging to choose one. Ron's business was struggling and I was disappointed that he had become somewhat paralyzed, was not following through on promises and was indecisive and overwhelmed. I still loved him but I couldn't authentically sing a mushy love song. John Scott suggested the song, "It Had to Be You" using Barbra Streisand's version. I fell in love with the song and the arrangement. I connected with its bittersweet vibe. To me, the song meant that despite your challenges and imperfections, I love you. That really fit what my heart was feeling at that point in time.

After our first rehearsal together had taken hours and was complicated, I was a bit nervous. John and Gio were struggling with harmonies for at least three of the songs, and our bass player was not jiving with Kurt. Yikes!!

John, Gio, Talia and I met a few more times on our own to work on harmonies; I couldn't figure out why John and Gio were still challenged; perhaps the harmonies were too complicated?

One of the highlights during the show was singing the meaningful yet upbeat Sara Bareilles song, "Many the Miles" with Talia, Gio and John doing backup vocals. It was the only time during the whole show that I let loose. The audience enjoyed it and I loved moving around the stage dancing, using my body and connecting with my backup singers. We also sang, "Rockin' Robin," "River of Dreams," and "Goodnight Sweetheart."

But then my Perfectionist's worst nightmare came true during the show when John and Gio wrestled with the lyrics while singing, "River of Dreams." It got worse when we sang "Good Night Sweetheart" and the harmonies were completely off. It was so bad that Kurt stopped playing because he didn't know what to play, so we were singing *a capella*. I was struggling to stay on key. Unfortunately, that was the final song before the encore.

We exited the stage and I was freaking out with a million emotions. My knee jerk reaction was anger towards John and Gio for screwing up. I was embarrassed that the audience had to experience such imperfection and at the same time I value my friendships and didn't want to make them feel bad. I knew John was feeling awful by the look on his face. I also was quite aware that in less than a minute, I needed to get back on stage and sing my final solo, "Grateful," a song about acknowledging and appreciating what we have in our lives.

*How was I going to sing that song authentically with all the turmoil I was experiencing?*

I didn't utter a word to John or Gio before returning to the stage. I took a deep breath, went back on stage, and told the audience:

*"Remember I mentioned earlier that my life has been a bit of a roller coaster ride? Kind of like our show this evening..."*

The audience laughed. Then I said,

*"Sometimes, I see the glass as half full or half empty.*
*Tonight I see it as three-quarters full.*
*May your cup runneth over."*

When I began to sing, I miraculously connected to my heart; it was my final moment to enjoy the show and connect to the audience. I sang about the challenges of life and gave thanks for what I have. That song held even more meaning for me at that time since that year had been incredibly challenging and I struggled to be present, aware and thankful for what WAS working in my life. I let all my struggles go and sang with all of my essence. I was proud of myself in that moment. That was the epitome of what "performing" means to me.

Surprisingly, I instantly released the horrible judgments and connected with my heart. I was authentic in acknowledging the challenges we experienced and that drew the audience more into the show. The thing that amazed me was that it was something I couldn't have planned for. The lesson? When I trust myself and stop trying to plan, my intuition and my Performer kicks in beautifully.

When the show was over, my Perfectionist quickly returned. Everyone went to sleep and I watched the show video gasping in horror as I viewed the screwed-up harmonies. I tortured myself by replaying the horrible scenes of the screw ups in my mind over and over again. I was challenged to let go of my judgment towards Gio and John. It was also interesting how John and Gio processed the situation. Gio accepted the screw ups as just a part of the process and didn't see it as a big deal. I admired her perspective yet, couldn't embrace that for myself. I could tell that John felt very badly and was beating himself up. I didn't want to make him feel any worse than he already did.

I felt sort of empty after that show as I analyzed what I had learned from the experience. I realized that I had complicated things. I created a difficult format with too many group numbers. Also, I should have started rehearsing earlier so that people could have more time to learn their parts. In addition, I had picked a musical director who was a fellow perfectionist! He has an amazing ear and is a great arranger but has a challenging time working with singers and other musicians. He seems to find everyone to be "not a professional" and below his standards. That is not the right match for me as it takes me to my own perfectionism. But boy, can he play piano!!

I am still figuring out what kind of show to do next. I like the idea of collaborating but I want to creatively express myself with simplicity and ease. I don't need to share the spotlight to justify my choices. But I do like having other singers in the show to help me entertain the audience, bring in a bigger crowd, provide diversity and frankly, help me lessen the load.

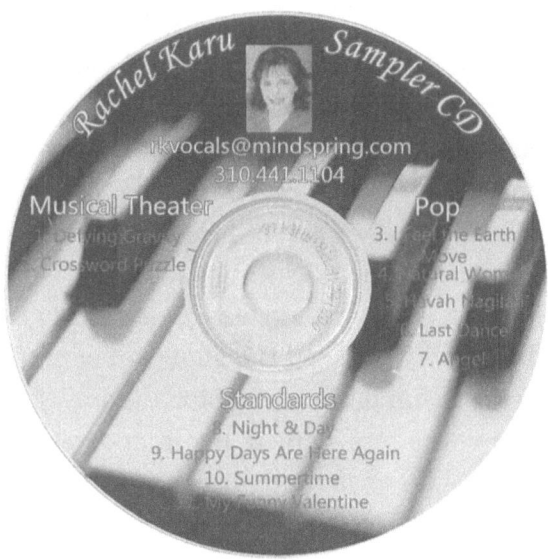

**Lessons Learned**

I learned that my deep rooted fear of abandonment and my desire to be liked sometimes causes me to hold back and not speak my truth. This can get me into deep trouble. I also realized how I was guilty of emotionally abandoning those close to me when we don't see eye to eye. The very behavior I despise in others. We are all mirrors for each other.

I continue to give myself permission and the freedom to follow my intuition when it comes to song choices and how I want to produce my shows. This is very empowering.

I started to reflect on and notice how much connection and intimacy I desire in relationships and when it makes sense to establish boundaries. This is an ongoing lesson.

**Deepen Your Learning**

1. How important is for you to be accepted or liked? Are you triggered when you do not believe you are being accepted or liked? If so, how do you know you are being triggered (e.g. What beliefs do you hold, where do you feel it in your body, what is your breathing like, etc.)?

   _____
   _____
   _____
   _____
   _____

2. Do you ever avoid discussing certain issues? What topics do you tend to avoid most? Does avoiding usually help or hinder the situation?

   _____
   _____
   _____
   _____
   _____

3. What type of spiritual rituals do you practice? How fulfilling are these practices?

   _____
   _____
   _____
   _____
   _____

4. How connected do you feel to your community (school, neighborhood, religious affiliation, etc.)? What can you do to deepen your connection?

_____
_____
_____
_____
_____

# 15
## No More Wheaties for Me!

As I mentioned earlier, around this time Ron decided he wanted to be his own boss and purchased a natural-stone restoration business, Marblelife. We borrowed money off the equity in our home to make this possible. The minute he stepped into his new role, I had a bad feeling that we would be fine for about two years until our money ran out and then he would be looking for another job. I just had a sense that this wasn't going to be a good fit for him.

Unfortunately my intuition was spot on and his business had been steadily declining (after just two years in business) and he came to the realization that we had to sell the business or risk going bankrupt! He also recognized that he needed to get a job (he signed an offer letter this week – yay!!). It is unfortunate that he came to these conclusions only after we got into debt and started struggling to pay our mortgage.

I suffered another blow on the physical front. After I had been bitching about taking a vacation to Cabo San Lucas with my parents and son Noam (without Ron and Talia), I wound up having a challenging trip for different reasons than expected: second degree burns on my arms and legs due to some sort of allergic reaction to the sun. I barely made it home, went on a dose of cortisone, and thought I was done with the whole mess.

But the next thing I knew, a new rash had developed and spread all over my body. I went to an allergist who informed me that the first round of medicine wasn't strong enough so he put me on a heavy dose of Prednisone (a nightmare drug!) for 15 days. He was so excited because he hadn't seen a systematic reaction like that since grad school. How cool...for HIM! He couldn't do the allergy tests to determine what caused the reaction until I finished the medication. In the meantime, he proclaimed,

*"You seem to be a highly allergic person so we need to do lots of allergy testing!"*

Dazed and amped up in Prednisone hell, I went for allergy tests without knowing what to expect. The nurse asked me to sit on a chair and put a pillow under my arms. She returned with the needle test. She poked me with needles to fill four panels on both my arms before casually delivering the following instructions as she left the room:

*"Sit for 20 minutes. Don't move."* and *"It may start to itch."*

The second she left, the tears started welling up. The last thing I wanted was more itching. I felt like a science experiment. I sat there struggling with how to comfort myself when I found myself quietly repeating "Om nava shivaya," the chant I learned in my meditation classes. I had never been able to make chanting a habit yet that is what came forward. After closing my eyes and continuing to chant for a while, I started to see a purple light in my head. I knew it was a good sign because I see purple whenever I am experiencing a relaxing or spiritual moment. I began to breathe and steady myself.

Then, after what seemed like an eternity, the doctor returned and informed me that I had some minor allergies to flowers, grass, trees, dogs and cockroaches (who knew?) before delivering the major bombshell: I am allergic to WHEAT! No problem – I just need to live in a bubble and change my entire way of eating. What could be next?

I left the office holding back tears, praying I would make it to my car without losing it. No wheat?? That was like a death sentence for me. I am an emotional eater and the little Rebel inside loves to eat whatever she wants. One of my most cherished pleasures had just been taken away.

As I got into the car, my thoughts were spinning. One voice was saying,

*You are going to be fine. You will do research on what you can eat. You will figure this out.*

At the same time, I was screaming and crying:

*How can this be happening to me?!* and *What did I do to deserve this?*

I started thinking about all the foods I could never eat again – like pizza (my all-time favorite), bread, pasta, cake...the list went on and on.

I called Ron and told him about my life sentence. In his usual rational way, he told me that I would be fine and it was no big deal. I told him:

*"I just found this out. Let me have my time to process this and my emotions."*

I mean, come on, give me a minute to be a victim, okay??

As soon as I got home, I logged onto the Trader Joe's website and looked up their gluten-free products – there were 16 pages of them! I scrolled through the list and began highlighting foods that interested me. Then, I began comparing ingredients to those the doctor said I couldn't have, just to be sure.

That evening I headed to Trader Joe's and began shopping. I started buying all kinds of foods I normally wouldn't buy just because I COULD! Chocolate and chips were allowable carbs! My Rebel was at play.

The next day, I met with my vegan friend Ivars who told me that my predicament was a blessing and that he couldn't wait to hear how I felt in a few months. Deep down, I knew that was probably true but I couldn't admit it in the moment.

After our meeting, I went across the street to Whole Foods. As I entered the market, I noticed the "Gluten-Free" shelves were marked with a big sign that was right in front of me. I gasped, stood still and looked at the large array of products. The tears surged, but happy ones this time. I had found my new home and experienced a sudden sense of hope. I realized that despite how bad I felt, everything was going to be okay. I traipsed down aisle after aisle (having abandoned the doctor's list at this point) in search of new food options.

One of the greatest moments was finding frozen cupcakes with this amazing looking frosting on top (I love frosting). After I spent a small fortune, I came home and couldn't wait to have dinner so I could enjoy my dessert. That first bite into the thawed cupcake was HEAVEN!! Right then, I knew I would find a way to deal with the situation. I might gain 100 pounds but I would be wheat-free. So, a day and a half after I thought my life as I knew it was over, I was able to embrace the change whole heartedly. Not a very long adjustment period, right?

**Lessons Learned**

Sometimes the best lessons arise from our worst experiences. The unexpected forces us to surrender to what is, change our perspective, and quickly embrace a new way of being. This is what happened to me when the universe informed me of my wheat allergy. I was proud of my resilience and my ability to quickly regroup. I couldn't continue eating wheat when I knew it was literally hurting me physically. I couldn't justify eating the cake or the pasta when I knew I would be in pain. Although this is challenging, it has been a blessing in disguise.

**Deepen Your Learning**

1. Reflect on a time you experienced what seemed like a tragedy and later turned into a blessing.

   _____
   _____
   _____
   _____
   _____

2. How did you initially react to the situation above? What process did you go through to shift your perception?

   _____
   _____
   _____
   _____
   _____

3. What did you learn about yourself during this life experience? How can you apply this to a current situation you are struggling with?

   _____
   _____
   _____
   _____
   _____

# 16
## This is Me in All My Glory

As the financial noose was slowly choking us, I learned to throw any fears related to my business out the window and really go for it. I no longer had the luxury of time to hope or wait to pursue my dreams.

I am now on a quest to integrate my creativity into my other work as a trainer and speaker. It started with identifying myself as a professional singer when being introduced to others. Then, my friend Jeanne had a wonderful idea to add a link to my email signature line that would let people hear me sing on YouTube. That really exposed my long-hidden secret of being a singer. People started approaching me to say that they had clicked on the link, and that they had no idea I was a singer. I also started singing at my professional training association's holiday parties; those certainly were "coming out" events for me.

Recently, I started incorporating singing into my training and speaking. It all began when I spoke at a CEO Association. Jay, the chairperson for the meeting, had clicked on my email signature and listened to my music. He complimented my voice and we talked about singing and the power of music.

The session I was to facilitate was on the topic of how to be a more effective coach and leader. Jay had nine CEOs in the room along with about 20 other people who reported to them. Jay introduced me as a singer; I told them if they asked me nicely, I might sing for them. At the end of the workshop, we gathered for lunch. I was not in a great mood since just before ending the session; one of the members complained that he wished I had focused more on the idea of setting effective goals. Setting goals didn't directly link to the coaching workshop I facilitated and he created a sour, awkward vibe in the room five minutes before ending the session. This is not the energy I want in the room seconds before they are about to complete an evaluation assessing me and the session. I was pretty annoyed.

As I was getting ready to leave, one of the members asked if I would sing. I felt the knot in my stomach forming. I was already angry and trying to keep my composure; now I was being asked to show more vulnerability by singing? But just at that moment, my "gentle strength" appeared. My intuition told me to shock them by being incredibly authentic. I decided to sing a verse from the beautiful, prayer-like song, "Grateful" that conveys the message that we need to be grateful for all we have even when life is rough. I sang it from my heart with conviction. It was like my soul was giving them the finger. I was saying in my heart,

> *Here is the real me. I am not full of shit, and I won't pretend to be someone I'm not to try to fit into your boy's club.*

I looked the CEOs in the eyes. Some felt uncomfortable while others were pleasantly shocked. They applauded and gave nice feedback, and then I went on my merry way.

Later, they emailed me their digital feedback on the entire session. Four out of the nine members felt that I should include my singing in my presentations. They said things like,

> *"Rachel, you were terrific."*
> *"I hope you will continue to include your singing in all your workshops."*

Wow! I had been thinking about that for years and pondering how to do it. Suddenly, the CEOs who had intimidated me were encouraging me to be creative and to share my gift. I had wrongly judged them for being stuck in their heads, theories and egos and now, they were giving me permission to shine in my authentic way from my heart. It was such a pleasant surprise to feel acceptance from people who I feared would not understand or appreciate me.

A few weeks later at a CEO session on the topic of "Leading Yourself and Others Through Change – How Self-Resilience Can Keep You Stable during Uncertain Times," I created a self-assessment that explored eight different competencies that comprise self-resilience (the ability to "bounce back" in the midst of change). I decided to sing a snippet of a song that related to the essence of each competency as I was defining it.

When I arrived to set up for the workshop, I had a strange calmness and feeling of eager anticipation to share my creative surprise with them. I had spent a lot of time finding songs to match each competency and had written out the lyrics to ensure that I wouldn't freak out if I forgot them. I was prepared to share my "gentle strength" with the world.

Once again, Larry, the meeting chairperson, introduced me as a singer. I immediately engaged the 14 male CEOs in the boardroom overlooking the golf course by having them stand up and sit down during some exercises to help them connect to the uncertain and uncomfortable feelings and thoughts that change can spark in us. After taking the self-assessment, they started opening up and addressing real issues that affected their professional and personal lives. Now it was time to define the eight competencies.

While they took the assessment, I was sucking on a cough drop and drinking a ton of water. I also went to pee, which is what I always do before singing (my little Perfectionist rituals were at play), before telling them the following:

> *"I invite you to look at the competency definition pages and to consider the thoughts and feelings that come up as we explore each competency in a unique way. The first one we will look at is self-awareness."*

I took another sip of water and took a deep breath. I closed my eyes and began singing a verse from "Defying Gravity" from the musical, "Wicked:"

*"I'm through accepting limits cause someone says they're so. Some things I cannot change but till I try, I'll never know. Too long I've been afraid of losing love I guess I'd lost. Well if that's love it comes at much too high a cost. I'd sooner buy defying gravity. Kiss me goodbye, I'm defying gravity. And you can't pull me down."*

I stood solid, with my feet planted on the ground. I looked them in the eye and stood in my power. I was declaring,

*Here I am! This is me in all my glory.*
*I accept me for who I am and that's all that matters.*

I could feel the silence and presence in that wonderful moment. I had everyone's complete attention. I ended the verse and — after a moment of silence – applause! I thanked them for their applause and shared my rationale for singing:

*"Number one, I am on a journey to integrate my creativity in all that I do. I am sick of compartmentalizing.*

*Number two, I want to get you out of your heads and hit you on a deeper level. Music connects us to our hearts."*

I took a deep breath and said,

*"And number three, in case you haven't noticed, I am modeling vulnerability when I sing. This takes a lot of courage. Some people have the misconception that being vulnerable is a weakness. I assert that it is extremely powerful to be vulnerable by standing grounded in your authenticity. It draws people in because they can relate to it; it gives others the freedom to be their authentic selves. You need to be vulnerable and authentic in order to be an effective coach and leader."*

I continued singing segments of songs that related to each competency. I could see some of the guys moving to the music. Some were even quietly singing along. That was a triumphant moment I will cherish forever.

Since that first step, I continued to sing at various speaking engagements and workshops I have facilitated. I am claiming my creativity and sharing it with CEOs, Human Resources professionals, and other leaders.

I had another wonderful experience speaking/singing at The Actors Fund, a wonderful organization that offers all types of social services to those in the entertainment industry – actors, camera people, directors, cinematographers, screenwriters, costumers, etc. A colleague who assists The Actors Fund with career services had asked me to speak. We decided I would facilitate a session called, "Create Your Career Marketing Plan – Take Charge of Your Career."

I had facilitated that session many times before but had customized it to match the participants' creative background. I arrived to a large sound stage with more than 150 people in the audience. Although I knew my material inside and out, I was a bit nervous knowing that I was talking to people in the entertainment industry (an industry I thought I wanted to be part of long ago). I had tapes playing in my head that recalled my rejection to my second year at the American Academy of Dramatic Arts; I was fighting my Gremlins.

I began speaking and emphasized the need to focus not only on our actions but on who we want to be at any given moment. I added a closed-eye visualization during which I asked them to recall a successful career-related experience whether it was a good audition, interview, networking event, etc. I asked them to recall:

*"Who were you being in that moment?*
*What was your mind set?*
*What kinds of thoughts were running through your brain?*
*How did your body feel?*
*What was your breathing like?"*

I asked them to capture those thoughts and feelings and to carry them forward during our workshop and when approaching any work-related events. I then told them:

*"Here is a perspective that assists me as it relates to my career."*

I took a deep breath and began to sing the first verse of "Defying Gravity" from "Wicked." When I stopped singing, there was a brief second of silence before…I heard the applause. I think I also heard an older man yell out,

*"Next!"*

I thought he had said it as if I had failed an audition but later, one attendee told me she thought he meant, "Encore!" My Gremlin wanted to hold onto the possible rejection but I quickly let it go. I still don't know if he actually said that or if it was my Gremlin desperately seeking something negative to affirm its judgments against me. I decided that it was probably a projection of his own experience auditioning and ignored his comment.

Then I shared with the audience my rationale for singing:

*"I am modeling vulnerability for you. There is tremendous strength in standing grounded in your authentic being – flaws and all. I am also sharing with you that everyone's career continues to evolve, even mine. I am now integrating my creative voice into my work in the business world — it can be done. You can be creative and work in corporate America."*

I continued the workshop and had so much fun. I wore a wireless microphone so I was able to walk up and down the aisles as participants completed exercises. They were engaged and the energy in the room was alive and exciting.

I ended the session by singing part of a John Buchinno song, titled "Taking the Wheel:"

*"I've been in the backseat long enough, tagging along for the ride.*
*I've been in the backseat long enough to know.*
*That you never get what you deserve if you never can decide.*
*There's only one way to get where you want to go...*
*Throwing down the pencil and grabbing a pen.*
*Taking the wheel, driving again.*
*Throwing down the pencil and writing in ink.*
*This is how I feel, this is what I think.*
*Dreaming again and making those dreams real.*
*Taking the wheel!"*

I raffled off 10 free coaching calls and as I wrapped up, crowds of people started approaching me. The feedback was overwhelmingly wonderful. Two people asked if I had a CD to sell (that affirmed that I need to produce a CD to be a companion to my book); two people approached me about editing my book; and numerous people shared how inspiring my story was and how much they appreciated my practical approaches to career management.

The Actors Fund session was an incredible milestone for me. I have been declaring my integrated self to the business world, letting them know that I sing. But that day, I owned my creativity and talent by letting the creative world know I was much more than a stuffy business woman. That was my "coming out party" to the creative world. What joy and power I experienced. It was a true success!

I had been trying for so long to mask my creativity and heart. But singing is the entryway to my soul so letting people hear my voice makes me extremely vulnerable. My intention and hope is that they will be touched on a deeper, more personal level, and that I will stand out in their eyes. Even if they don't remember my topic, they will remember the speaker who sings.

I am also very excited about finishing this book and creating a one-person show during which I will sing snippets of songs that fit different key moments of my story. I enrolled in a writing class and had the chance to do, two ten-minute performances. The response was amazing. People told me that they felt my authenticity and vulnerability, that they were touched, and that I made them feel on a deeper level. That was exactly what I was going for. It was also so freeing for me to share my story without any big production, and just to sing from my heart.

I also plan to create a keynote presentation that utilizes my story, and to present it at conferences. The quest to integrate continues; my vision is gaining clarity and the feedback I am receiving is so affirming. My new challenge is to make money by expressing myself and, boy, do I need to make money fast.

**Lessons Learned**

The idea of integrating all my various aspects of myself came alive for me at last and my work and personal world began to interconnect. This was a huge step for me as it required my willingness to be vulnerable and trust my voice and creativity – my gentle strength.

I had an inner knowing and the strength to follow my intuition regardless of any judgment from others and the outcome I accomplished. This was a bold step which was largely inspired by my life circumstances. This was "do or die" time. I looked fear straight in the eye and moved forward. It was so empowering to accept myself and my gifts without relying too heavily on external validation. I knew I could deliver the goods in a creative, unique way!

**Deepen Your Learning**

1. **How compartmentalized is your life currently?**

_____
_____
_____
_____
_____

2. **How can you integrate more of your values and passions into various life areas?**

3. **What valuable blind spots have you unearthed as a result of feedback you have received?**

4. **Who can you seek feedback from right now to help your growth?**

5. **When was the last time you were vulnerable? How did you feel? What was the impact?**

# 17
## You Know You Make Me Want to Shout!

Another opportunity to stretch my creative muscles happened when my friend Lori hired me to provide the entertainment for her law firm's thirtieth anniversary party. Lori had been to some of my cabaret shows and has been a huge champion of my talent; I was so flattered when she offered me the opportunity to put together a band for her big event.

My Perfectionist Gremlin made a brief visit after Lori had first asked if I was interested, saying,

*You don't have a band. How can you put a four-hour event together? You've never done this before!*

A lovely list of excuses. But my Performer kicked in pretty quickly, and recognized I could hire a professional band and be the lead singer.

Synchronicity was definitely at play as I had met a kind and wonderful band leader Larry about six months prior at a friend's Bar-Mitzvah party. I was so impressed by him that I wanted to meet him, and did. Not long after that, I was asked to sing the National Anthem and Hatikvah (the Israel National Anthem) at our synagogue's annual dinner dance (a big 300-attendee event). It so happened that Larry's band was the entertainment for the evening, so we were able to meet beforehand and practice the songs; I also gave him my demo tape. We had an immediate connection and have been friendly ever since. I asked Larry if he would back me up at the lawyer's event and he graciously agreed.

That type of event was a big stretch for me and was an opportunity for my Perfectionist and my Performer to duke it out. As I mentioned previously, when I create and perform cabaret shows, my Perfectionist tries to organize and control everything to ensure success. I plan the sequencing of the songs, the "patter" in between songs, and all the other details. Larry likes to work the energy of the room and call out songs as we go. He also doesn't rehearse; it freaked me out at first.

*How can I perform without rehearsing?*
*How will I know all the songs?*

I authentically shared my fears and concerns with Larry. He told me to create a song list and songbook for him and Charlie the piano player. He also told me that I could have a music stand with all my music ready to go and that I didn't have to memorize all the songs. What a concept! I pondered this notion for weeks.

*Would my Perfectionist Gremlin give me permission to glance at the lyrics as I was singing?*

After much contemplation, I embraced the idea.

Talia's boyfriend lent me a music stand and I decided to create a lyrics book so I wouldn't have to sort through sheet music. I also painstakingly created the two music books for the musicians. That took hours to figure out; I needed to make two-sided copies and tape the music to help the musicians do less page flipping. I got so frustrated at one point that I could barely take it anymore. Ron spent hours helping me; it had become a family project.

Larry was gracious enough to come to my home with his guitar and we played music together. What an incredible experience! I felt very comfortable with him and he really liked my voice. The notion of rehearsing with the pianist then surfaced. I told him:

*"There are some new songs that I really need to work on and I would prefer to rehearse them with Charlie rather than someone else."*

He gave this some thought and spoke to Charlie. They finally agreed to both meet me for a rehearsal at my parents' house since they had a baby-grand piano. He asked that I pay $25 for gas money — what a steal!!

The pieces were all coming together beautifully until I got sick. I wasn't sure I would have a voice for the show. I had to postpone our precious rehearsal because I couldn't sing. But when we finally met, it was pure heaven. My voice was just starting to heal and I was so grateful that it held out for our two-hour rehearsal. It felt wonderful to be playing with professional musicians who were patient, talented and sensitive to playing the arrangements the way I desired.

The night before the big event, I had a major stomachache. Something from dinner hadn't agreed with me and I was in the bathroom a few times during the night. I woke up early, exhausted to take my son Noam to his 9:00 a.m. basketball game (Noam is really becoming a wonderful player, and it is incredible to see his confidence and skill level grow). We returned home, ate lunch and I took an hour's nap.

Then, it was off to Bobbie Brown's shop to have my makeup done — I love the woman, Lauren, who works there. She does an incredible job without pressuring me to buy products. Of course, I always do purchase something small but leave feeling her talent was way worth my minimal investment.

After returning home, I changed and Ron and I dropped the kids off at my parents'. He drove me to Shutter's, a fancy, Santa Monica boutique hotel where the event was being held. I warmed up my voice with vocal exercises and drank hot tea with lemon and honey on my way over. Ron returned home and planned to meet us later to tape the event. When I found the room, Larry the bandleader was already there sweating up a storm. He had taken on the challenge of schlepping all of his equipment using the service elevator. I helped him the best I could, but there wasn't much for me to do. It was a small, elegant room; the highlight was that we were overlooking the ocean. It had been raining earlier in the day so there was a beautiful display of white-and-dark-colored clouds resting over the crashing waves.

I asked the hotel staff if I could get some dinner delivered before the event. While I waited, I wanted to set intentions for the evening but I had so much nervous energy, it was hard to focus. I started writing out intentions on a piece of paper while talking to Larry (not very effective), when Ernetsto from the hotel returned with my food. They showed up with a loaf of bread and a big, yummy plate of spaghetti! I felt badly but I told him,

> *"My apologies but I am allergic to wheat and I cannot eat this. Could you possibly bring me a salad with some protein?"*

He looked a bit surprised and showed up about 15 minutes later with a Cobb Salad drenched in dressing with avocado and hardboiled egg (I dislike both immensely). I just said,

> *"This is great, thank you."*

It was strange to me that he didn't ask what I wanted but, instead, had the staff decide what they thought was appropriate. I rummaged through the salad picking out the chicken and trying to ignore the hardboiled egg. At least I ate some protein that would hold me over for the big event.

Afterwards, Charlie the piano player arrived. We talked for a while and I helped him get situated. I then struggled attempting to figure out how to set up my music stand and have the microphone close enough so people could hear me. At that point, Ron showed up and he helped me with this. My Perfectionist was definitely at play as I was setting up. I was thinking of what was needed for every possible turn of events. I shoved cough drops into the lyrics book just in case. I found a way to balance my bottle of water on the music monitor next to me. On the ledge behind me, overlooking the ocean, I placed another bottle of water, tissues, a pen, and my lip pencil, lipstick, and lip gloss. I also placed my giant purple backpack on the floor nearby just in case I needed something else. I was set.

I went into the bathroom to change into my outfit and my "four-hour heels" (which is about the maximum I can stand), and transform into the Performer. I took my time as I put on my Jackie-O black skirt suit with a classy top, skirt and jacket with a pretty, ruffled color. I touched up my makeup; put on perfume, rubbed sesame oil on my legs to help them shine, and finally, perched myself upon the dreaded heels. I looked at myself in the mirror and thought to myself,

*You are ready for this. You look great!*

I took a deep breath, looked myself in the eye and recited my affirmations:

*"I am a freedom flyer, surrendering to the flow of now, loving trusting, and accepting myself and you. I am a beautiful, trusting, authentic woman freely sharing my truth; Peacefully receiving and giving love."*

I was excited and a bit nervous yet, I had an inner knowing that everything was going to be alright. I was ready for the challenge.

I returned to the room and could hear that guests were entering the adjacent room where cocktails were being served. It was now 6:15 and the doors to the party room would open at 7 o'clock. Our drummer Dave had yet to show up, and it was making me nervous. Larry and Charlie told me that he usually shows up just moments before the gig, and that everything always works out well. But I started to get concerned; Charlie assured me that he had a drum kit on his electric keyboard if we needed it as a backup, and that put my mind at ease.

Dave showed up around 6:30 while Larry was changing and Charlie was having a smoke. Ron and I helped him set up. Dave seemed very relaxed and I could tell that he liked to tell stories. That was our first meeting, so I recounted how I had met Larry, and that I had hired him for this gig and not the other way around. I wanted him to know who was the boss for the evening!

It was 7 o'clock before I knew it, and people started entering the room. We were waiting for my friend Lori to tell us when they wanted me to introduce the partners so they could give a toast. The band started playing instrumental music and, immediately, my fear set in. I thought I had to pee (even though I had just gone about 20 minutes before), but the panic had set in and I was thinking,

*"How long will I have to stand here and sing before I can go to the bathroom again?"*

I debated what to do. Finally, I told Charlie that I would be right back.

*"No problem,"* he said.

I ran to the bathroom (which, thankfully, was very close to the party room) and afterwards, I started shaking my hands out to let out the nervous energy. I re-entered the room ready to do this!

After a couple of instrumentals, Larry called out,

*"This Masquerade"* for me to sing.

Of course, we had never rehearsed that song and, I hadn't sung it in more than 20 years. Luckily, we had checked the key while setting up our equipment. I found the page in my lyric book and thought,

*Okay, here we go...*

The room was buzzing with chatter and I could feel the excited energy in the air. I listened to the song's opening and began the song. Being a bit nervous, I wasn't singing with full voice. I kept looking at the lyrics to make sure I remembered them. People would glance at me and then continue talking — that was actually a relief. I started to ease into the role of party entertainer. As I sang, I got more comfortable. I remembered the recorded version of the song, so I knew when the band would want to do an instrumental. They came in right on cue. The song flowed and worked well — yay!

*One song down and many more to go.*

In addition to being the singer, I was also the master of ceremonies. I invited the senior partners to the microphone to make toasts. As the partners were acknowledging employees, the band was right on cue hitting the drum or making music to acknowledge people. This band was very professional and they knew exactly what they were doing. Larry started calling out different songs. The other band members sang as well. So when they sang a song that I wasn't involved in, I swayed to the music. Sometimes I would add backup vocals and harmonize with them. That was fun. It also gave me the opportunity to suck on a cough drop and then replace it in the paper wrapper before I sang again. It was fun not always having to be the center of attention.

Then, Lori and another law partner decided to make an unexpected toast. It was wonderful to be a fly on the wall and see Lori in her professional role. She talked about the challenges of returning to work after having her two boys, and how much she enjoyed working with the other attorneys and support staff at the firm. I was touched, and it was inspiring to hear Lori authentically share from her heart. She wasn't putting on a persona; she wasn't pretending like she didn't have a family or a life. She candidly shared the struggles of balancing a very full life. I was so proud and grateful to have her as my friend. It confirmed that she was one of my tribe.

As the party continued, Lori asked if two of the attorneys could sing a song.

*"Sure,"* I responded.

Two nicely dressed attorneys approached us and I was ready to hand over the microphone. One of them asked Larry if he could play his guitar. Larry graciously handed it over. He had a shocked look on his face like,

*What are we in for?*

The attorney began playing "Something" by the Beatles and the other attorney, who was quite tipsy, attempted to sing. He didn't know the words to the song and he kept flipping through my lyric book to find the words. I told him,

*"You won't find them there. This isn't a karaoke book."*

The whole scene was quite entertaining, and the partygoers were getting into what was happening. Once the duo had completed their song, I began singing Alanis Morrisette's "Hand in Pocket." The tipsy, good-looking attorney in the tuxedo stood next to me and we sang a duet. It was hysterical. We started adding hand motions that illustrated the song like "high-fiving" each other, holding up our fingers in a peace sign, and motioning like we were flicking a cigarette. The funniest moment for me was when we got to the lyric that said,

*"I'm brave but I'm chicken shit."*

I wasn't planning on saying "shit." I pointed to the word, "shit" right before we sang the lyric and the attorney continued to shout out the profanity while I stood silent. Too funny.

I sang all types of music including "Night and Day," "Chain of Fools," "If I Ain't Got You," "I Feel the Earth Move," and "My Funny Valentine." As I warmed up, I became more comfortable and my voice started to soar. I was noticing the partygoers more and they were beginning to notice me as well.

Suddenly, after I started to sing "Smooth Operator," there were people on the dance floor. That cracked me up as I had never sung that song before and it wasn't particularly one of my favorites. I kept glancing at my lyrics book trying to see the words and look at the audience. After we finished, Larry told the audience:

*"We are now going to sing one of 'R.K.'s requests."*

I piped up with,

*"That's me"*

And we went into "The Lion Sleeps Tonight." You might recall that fun song that starts with

*"Aweema weh, aweema weh"*

The next thing I knew, the dance floor was full and people were singing along. Larry motioned that we would extend the song since people were into it. I looked at Larry and Charlie for guidance as to where we would go with the song. That was such an exciting high to see people enjoying the song without my knowing exactly where we were headed next.

Just before we ended the other song, Larry called out,

*"Shout!"*

Then Dave, our drummer, started singing,

*"You know you make me want to shout."*

I started singing with him and raising my hand in the air when we sang,

*"SHOUT!"*

More and more people were on the dance floor, and Dave stopped the song to ask more to join in and dance.

He continued to drum when he started going a little overboard saying things like,

*"We haven't asked a lot of you up until this point. We didn't ask you to carry our instruments in the rain. We won't ask you to tear down our equipment when we are done."*

At that point, I became a little uncomfortable. I quietly said into the microphone:

*"I think they get the point."*

He went on for a good three minutes until finally, he came back to the song as the partygoers danced away, having a great time. I sang and danced with them. When Dave asked for audience participation, I acted as if I was a participant and sang their parts and danced too. I was having a blast and I was thrilled that everyone was dancing! That was the highlight of the night for me.

Larry decided to call a break after that song. My intuition told me that wasn't a great time for a break and, unfortunately, I was correct. After we returned from the break, people started leaving and moving back to the bar area. Lori said we should keep playing, so we just kept going until we were basically playing for ourselves. I asked Larry if we could sing, "Let's Fall in Love." I had never sung it in public, but I had worked on it quite a bit. As I sang, Lori and her husband Kirk started dancing. It was such a joy serenading them. They are lovely people and wonderful friends. Jay, the senior partner, and his wife were gathering their coats to leave but when they heard me singing, they put down their coats and began to dance. Oh, that was a precious moment – singing a love song for two dancing couples. What a great way to end a magical evening!

We packed up our things and said goodbye to the band members. And then my Rebel was ready to play! I usually like to have a drink or two after getting wired from the adrenaline flow. Ron and I got the car from the valet and started driving down Ocean Blvd. towards Venice. We started brainstorming about where to go, and I remembered a cool seafood restaurant we had eaten at years ago. We drove and drove and couldn't find it. While we were looking for the restaurant, I noticed a great coffee and breakfast place, so we headed back there. We had a lovely time talking about the evening while I was drinking a decaf non-fat latte and eating a chicken pesto salad. I was actually on such a natural high that I didn't feel deprived not having my drink. I went to bed around 1 a.m., which is very early for me when I perform. I normally cannot get to sleep until much later.

The whole experience was a blast, and I was left pondering how to do more of these gigs. Less rehearsal, fewer expenses, and I don't have to market it to get people to show up. I get paid more; I help musicians make good money, and I am truly entertaining folks. Who could ask for anything more??

I was thinking about where to advertise the band, and that I must talk to Larry about including him in my marketing. I figured he would be quite happy if I were to bring him work, so that shouldn't be an issue. I was so excited to see where it all might lead.

## Lessons Learned

It was incredibly affirming to sing at a party with a band, entertain the audience, and make money!! What a high!

There was so much learning from this experience. I trusted that I could be successful when accepting the opportunity. I worked with professional musicians and asked for what I needed to be triumphant. I felt incredibly free and relaxed when I surrendered my need for perfection by allowing myself to use a lyrics book during the event. I felt like I was fulfilling my destiny on my terms.

## Deepen Your Learning

1. **What expectations do you currently place on yourself that aren't serving you?**

   _____
   _____
   _____
   _____

2. **Where can you release or modify expectations of yourself and/or others so you can experience greater joy?**

   _____
   _____
   _____
   _____

3. Describe an experience where you knew you were fulfilling your destiny?

   _____
   _____
   _____
   _____

4. Are there any areas or situations happening in your life where you can relinquish control?

   _____
   _____
   _____
   _____

# 18
## Reality Song: What are the Lessons and Can I Learn Them Already?!

I am in the eye of the storm. I am at the center watching the dangling particles of my life swarm around me. Sometimes I am solid and grounded as I observe all the swirling factors. Other times I am sucked into the storm and feel like I am in a tornado being thrown into unknown territory, waiting to crash to the ground.

It feels like the world is caving in on me: financial pressures, health issues, challenges getting my singing off the ground. What am I supposed to understand from all of this? I keep moving forward, holding my head up high, doing what I need to do to generate business, fulfill my dreams, and be a responsible mother, wife, daughter, friend, etc. It seems like I am being hit from all directions:

- I try to modify our home loan, and I get a foreclosure notice (just writing the words gives me a knot in my stomach)
- I am networking like a maniac, and yet no business has cropped up
- Ron's business is failing and we need to decide if we are going to dissolve it or hand it over to my dad to run
- My daughter Talia's Bat Mitzvah is in a week, and I still haven't learned my Torah portion. Plus the financial strain of it all is painful!
- I get a singing gig at Hadassah, and it gets cancelled

- I invite Gio to be part of a singing gig I get at Roxbury Park, and she bails out because there's too little time and it's too much pressure on us
- I finally post some videos of me singing on YouTube, and my piano player demands I take them down or edit him out

I have been sitting with these realities for many weeks; it is a surreal feeling. I go on living my regular life – taking care of the kids, seeing friends, trying to build my business, applying for full-time jobs (yuck), and strategizing how to incorporate more singing in my life. Everything seems normal. But I know it is far from normal! I know that at any point, the rug can be pulled out from us. I know that I am about to make some of the biggest and toughest decisions I have ever made.

This feeling was reinforced when I was having lunch with a friend and a homeless man burst into the middle of the crowded restaurant screaming at the top of his lungs that he was tired and that he wanted the restaurant to call the police so he could go to jail to get a shower, a hot meal, and a bed. I sat there silently, in absolute shock. The episode continued for about 10 minutes but it felt like an eternity. I suddenly noticed that I was crying. I was petrified by the idea that I could become that homeless person and be on the street. My friend looked at me, mortified, not knowing what to say. I did my best to explain my fear and she tried to reason with me saying that it won't happen to me. She struggled to understand the anxiety and discomfort I had endured for so long.

Many of our friends are upper-middle class and I felt awkward sharing our woes with them. I was a bit embarrassed and concerned that they wouldn't relate to our challenges. As I continued to open up to my inner circle, I felt blessed by the love and support we felt from our friends even if their circumstances were different. We all have our unique obstacles to overcome.

As mentioned above, we have been attempting to get a loan modification on our home for a year now, and the process drags on. We haven't paid our mortgage for about eight months and have destroyed our credit. And I was always the girl who paid her credit card in full! The reality of the situation makes me sick. I hate the fact that we cannot afford our mortgage and that we are not being responsible about making our payments.

What had eaten away at me for many months was the reason we could not afford our mortgage: Ron had taken out a loan against our mortgage to start his (now-failed) business. After going through an emotional rollercoaster-ride of feelings – denial, anger, resentment (which still ebb and flow), I am more in acceptance of "what is," and I am so happy that Ron has found a job that pays base salary plus commission.

The attorney keeps saying :

*"two more weeks until we know if you will be approved for the loan modification..."*

Well, two weeks turned into too many months. Ron's parents offered to pay the mortgage to help us avoid foreclosure, which was amazing and terribly uncomfortable for me. I hate having to ask them for money. Ron wants to hold off on paying the mortgage for a few more months to see if we get our loan modification. His rationale is that once we are approved, the outstanding balance will be incorporated into the loan so it is a waste to pay it now. My parents are freaking out and asking why we aren't paying it. I am torn right down the middle.

The likelihood is that we might not be able to afford a modified loan even if we are approved. Then, we would have two big decisions in our laps: One, do we declare bankruptcy or attempt a debt consolidation? Again I notice that just writing the word "bankruptcy" makes me sick to my stomach. And, two, if we sell our home, do we move to an apartment in a less expensive part of L.A., such as the San Fernando Valley, or do we use the profit from selling our home to fulfill Ron's dream to make a clean start moving to Israel? But I wonder,

*Would moving to Israel really be a clean start?*

I am so challenged by this decision. I could make a case for Ron and the kids to move there, but what about me? I am having a hard time separating this decision from my previous negative experiences there. I also realize that some of the challenges of living in Israel are simply that – *my* challenges. And they are my challenges wherever I may reside.

I have done my best to seek support and tackle the various internal layers that can help me make these monumental decisions. My husband and I have been seeing a therapist to talk about many issues. It has been helpful for a third party to help Ron take a look at himself. I am not going to run to Israel only to find that he is still not happy and fulfilled because he hasn't really done any self-reflection. I think he has an unrealistic expectation or fantasy that being near his family will solve his insecurities and self-doubt.

I have continued working with both my coach and my therapist in an attempt to sort out my feelings and thoughts regarding Israel. Some of these thoughts and feelings are irrational. I am extremely triggered when I go to Israel; it brings out a primitive, deep-down fear of being abandoned. I feel that Ron gets sucked into the *"borg"* (his family) and that I am alone on some desert island praying he will come back.

I have been exploring how my troubled relationship with Ron's dad is a mirror for other relationships in my life. I so want to feel a part of groups whether it be family, synagogue or work and yet, I also want to have my independence. It has been challenging for me to set boundaries without horrible feelings of guilt. I have been conditioned to feel that I am being selfish unless I am continually in service to the group or the collective. These feelings come to a head when I am in Israel. I also see how Ron's dad is similar to my own parents. They both hold many expectations, rules and regulations about what is proper and "right."

In the past, I have become like an amoeba trying to conform to everyone's desires and rules. But that comes with a price.

It sparks my rebellious side and my resentment grows. Eventually, I disconnect from those people because I am sick of battling them, and I am done being whoever they think I should be. So instead of speaking my authentic truth and staying grounded in who I am, I separate from them and hide. Of course, they sense my distance and are baffled by it. My fear has me separating from them versus confronting them because I am afraid they will leave me or hate me. The truth is that if they have already emotionally abandoned me, what do I have to lose? But if I don't stand up to them, I will lose my identity and my soul.

I long for others' acceptance and love, but the truth is that I must love and accept myself. That is the most important love to experience. I have a favorite tree in my neighborhood that I named, "Glory." She is a beautiful magnolia tree that takes up a huge corner. I love her roots because they are coming out of the ground, exposed for the world to see. She is powerful and strong while being vulnerable. She has the most amazing and abundant branches. When she is in bloom, she is fragrant with her white flowers. She is generous and a good hostess to the birds that she lets nest high up in her branches. I spoke to the owner of the home where Glory resides, and she told me that she bought the house because she loved the tree. She told me how her now-grown kids used to play on that tree and that, years later, her daughter had climbed it in her wedding dress.

I am learning to develop a backbone like the trunk of that large tree. I can see myself with my roots solidly planted in the ground. My roots are slightly visible so I am vulnerable, but I know that I am solidly connected to the earth. Nothing can shake my foundation. I am still learning to "fill the well" from within instead of seeking others to fill it for me; my progress waivers back and forth. It is a journey, right?

I have been struggling to remember how I once felt about Israel. I loved the freedom I had experienced there. I enjoyed the nightlife. I valued living in a Jewish country knowing that most people have a common bond with me. But now, I view it with uneasiness - being with Ron's family and feeling so different and alone.

*What am I supposed to do?*

I asked God and I heard,

*"Get a job."*

I don't know if it was truly the voice of God (if there is a God), or if it was my parents' voices that are so fucking engrained in my head. I have bonded with my Gremlin and I cannot seem to shake its grip at the moment.

It is hard to believe that all of these challenges would be resolved upon my simply getting a job. Instead, I see new challenges arising like,

*Who is going to pick up my kids after school?*
*Who will be with them during the Jewish holidays?*
*When will I have any time to pursue my singing?*

The thought of being in an office five days a week, sitting in a chair, having to justify my existence and quantify my efforts seems like death to me. I have been there, done that, and I don't want to go back.

It brings up the theme I just mentioned about craving a sense of belonging, yet still wanting my independence. I want to feel part of the department, aligned with the company mission. But then there is a part of me that says,

*Fuck you!*

I want to help people and the company because I truly care, not because I will be viewed as an outcast if I don't. I want to use my creativity to have impact on things I find meaningful, not because it is being dictated by the corporation. I want to have the flexibility to come and go as I please and not have to write down my hours or feel like someone is looking over my shoulder.

In spite of my resistance, I sent out my resume to about 15 headhunters yesterday seeking both part-time and full-time employment. We shall see. I have no desire for an office job AND I don't want to lose my home. It's is a difficult decision to make.

Everything feels hard, painful, and fearful. I feel the anxiety, anger, and resentment all building up inside of me. I hear myself thinking,

*I kind of wish I could have a nervous breakdown and just be so dysfunctional that everyone would need to figure things out without me.*

On some level, I don't want to be part of the game anymore. I have given it my all and it doesn't seem to be enough, so count me out. I wish I could be a helpless victim. I wish, I wish. I know that isn't possible and that the universe is calling on me to be even more present, aware, and active. I feel like the universe is dragging me somewhere kicking and screaming. I had a dream the other night that I was at the bottom of a large dugout dirt circle and that people at the top of the circle are shooting at me. I am dodging the bullets, running in the circle, and barely staying alive. That is how my life feels. Like I'm barely making it...barely, barely, barely.

How am I supposed to serve others and motivate them if I am *barely* making it? It makes me feel like a fraud, an imposter. Of course, I know that's my perfectionism but it does make me wonder if my strategy is off. Maybe we are all supposed to be drones, living in a corporate box; bringing home the paycheck; only caring about our kids and family. And society seems to expect the drones to be dead inside. We are not supposed to have a passion; we are not supposed to take care of ourselves and reach for the stars. But how can that be? It goes against every fiber of my being.

*What are the lessons here?*
*What am I supposed to do?*

I pray that I will receive the answers quickly before my home is taken away from me.

It is now less than two weeks before the official foreclosure begins. The mortgage company called me two weeks ago to tell me that our modification request had been denied. Our new attorney says that the case isn't closed and submitted our modification request to his friend at our bank. I pray this will work. The attorney tells me not to worry until we hear back from his connection.

Sometimes, this surreal existence reminds me of when I was in college. I always felt the silent pressure of having many assignments due and tests to prepare for. The pressure was constantly on my shoulders and, even though I had fun, I couldn't completely relax knowing I had business to take care of.

I am still asking myself,

*What are the lessons?*

One theme that comes forward is that I need to actively engage in life – even the unpleasant aspects of it. I need to face my fears and not rely on Ron.

This uncertainty has brought some new perspective. I have been pushed into taking more risks and into owning my life. That has inspired more creativity and juiciness in my life. If not for the whole financial nightmare and needing to decide whether or not we are moving to Israel, life would actually be quite meaningful and enjoyable.

So I have now laid out the story and all its tactical components. The emotional part is rocky and feels like a roller coaster with steep valleys that make me want to vomit. Some days I am strong and clear. Other days, I am confused and scared. Some days I am angry with Ron for getting us into this mess. And then I'm angry with myself for allowing this to happen. I am annoyed that, despite all my efforts and hard work, I am not making enough money.

*But here is what I am proud of:*

1) I have been honest and open with my friends and colleagues about my situation.

2) I have asked for help and assistance even though it is extremely uncomfortable.

3) I have held my head high and have kept moving forward. I have been perpetually proactive in seeking new business and in strategizing how to get out of this situation.

4) I have been honest with my daughter Talia about the situation. I only hope that I have not instilled too much fear in her.

5) I have continued to do fun things and enjoy life. I have used this as an opportunity to reach out to friends and appreciate the simpler aspects of life.

6) I am writing about this unpleasant journey despite my embarrassment and pain. Somehow, I will turn my mess into a message that will inspire others.

There is no room for perfectionism in my current situation. I am being forced to surrender to what is, to accept, and move on. I am learning how to live and love myself despite apparent failures all around me. Could this be the lesson I was supposed to learn?

**Lessons Learned**

I once again realized there are many lessons to be gained from any situation, especially adversity. It seems we keep receiving the same lessons over and over again until we truly "get it."

One thing I absolutely know about myself is that I am uncomfortable being in limbo. I also learned that when the chips are down, I will do everything in my power to succeed. I throw all fear out the window and take charge. I let my Performer take the lead. I thrive in the face of fear and adversity. It is comforting to know that I can trust this aspect of myself.

**Deepen Your Learning**

1. Think of a current struggle or challenge. What lessons are being presented to you to learn?

   _____
   _____
   _____
   _____

2. How do you feel and behave when you are in limbo?

   _____
   _____
   _____
   _____

3. What messages do you give yourself about how to experience life? Examples include: "it's all good," "go with the flow," "I am barely getting by" or, "life is hard and I must work hard." How do these messages impact your thoughts, feelings, and actions?

   _____
   _____
   _____
   _____

# 19
## Living My Dream All Along

I felt like I was coming down with something during an intensive two-day business trip to Houston. It started with a strange sensation in my chest and a little cough but I felt that I was doing okay and even sang during both sessions. After one of them, I had a face-to-face meeting with a new coaching client from Texas, and then met my cousin Jane for dinner. I was productive, active, and busy.

But while driving to the airport, my cough had increased and I began to have a strange sensation like I was coming down with the plague. By the time I landed in Los Angeles, I was achy and feverish.

On my first night home, my cough was getting worse and my head was cloudy. I honored my 10 a.m. coaching call primarily because I felt comfortable enough with that client to tell her I wasn't well. I coached her while lying in bed and we actually had a very productive session.

Now, the big question was: should I keep my 1–3 p.m. face-to-face session at my home with a 360-degree feedback debrief using an assessment that was new to me? That would mean my having to prepare for the session and clean up my house. I realized that I would not be at my best in that state so I apologetically cancelled my session. My client was gracious and we rescheduled.

I called my doctor and was relieved when he prescribed some medicine over the phone. Doctor's office visits can be costly and I honestly could not afford his care at that time. I took the medicine and it helped slightly.

That night, I barely slept due to my terrible dry cough. I tried to sleep with my head propped up but that made my neck extremely tight and achy. My increasing fever only added to my discomfort. As the cough worsened, I fretted,

*I am losing my voice with each cough!*

I had a band rehearsal for my first big event gig in four days.

*Would I make it?*

I needed to get up at 5:15 a.m. the next morning to kick off the monthly training association meeting I led. I awoke feeling completely groggy and my head was spinning. My throat was killing me, my whole body was aching and quivering, and I had a 102-degree temperature. But I was determined to at least kick off the meeting. I told myself that I wouldn't stay long.

So I got up, dressed professionally and did my makeup. I had to at least appear normal, right? I drove to the Whole Foods store (where I held the meetings) and discovered that the room wasn't set up properly.

*"Noooo,"* I groaned.

That meant I would have to move large tables and chairs. I was praying that someone else would arrive to help. A few moments later, Jim, the Whole Foods manager, showed up. He was happy to help and I told him he had

*"...answered my prayers."*

He replied,

*"It is so great to be the answer to someone's prayer."*

People began to trickle in, and one of the participants offered to make my announcements for me so that I could go home. Although I hated missing the meeting, I was grateful for his offer. I said, "Hello" to folks and was careful not to kiss them. I made my rounds and then promptly excused myself. My duty was done.

I headed home to prepare for my next challenge – an interview with my daughter and husband for a potential high school. We had been waiting months for the meeting and I wanted to be there. On my way home, I stopped at the drug store and found a stronger form of Mucinex. Praying it would work, I took the pill. But after awhile, my head began to spin. I was so dizzy; I was wondering how I could make it. I asked Ron to drive. He wasn't thrilled about that since he had a meeting afterwards in the opposite direction. I told him,

*"I might not make it if I drive"* and he agreed.

Before we left, I started feeling the full effects of the medicine. Something was not agreeing with me and I felt sick to my stomach; I ran to the bathroom.

By the time we picked Talia up from school and arrived at the high school, I felt like I was in a surreal nightmare. I could barely speak. I was coughing and running to the bathroom every five minutes. Talia was the first to go in and speak with the admissions director. While we were waiting for our turn, a parent-docent appeared to say she would be taking us on a tour after the interview. I thought, there is no way I will survive a tour. She must have been reading my non-verbal language when she suggested,

*"We can always reschedule the tour."*

I thought,

*Is it really necessary to take the tour again?*

Talia and I had already toured the campus and I could not imagine scheduling another thing into my life at that time.

A moment later, the admissions director appeared. I declined to shake her hand, letting her know I was quite ill. She quickly offered,

*"Talia can take the tour while I speak with you."*

I was so grateful for her offer. We entered her office and she told us she wasn't feeling well, either, due to morning sickness. I congratulated her. We had a very pleasant meeting despite the fact that I felt like I was in a drug-induced fog. Luckily, my stomach held up during our talk.

Once home, I was pretty useless. My cough worsened and a rash appeared on both arms. No doubt I was allergic to one of the medications I took. My skin is so sensitive; I couldn't risk the rash getting worse so I decided to not take either medication. That night, I snuggled in bed and dozed off for a few minutes before the coughing began. I couldn't stop. I didn't want to wake Ron so I moved to the lounge chair in the living room, put a blanket over me, and attempted to sleep. I continued to cough throughout the night without relief. With every cough, I thought:

*My voice is dying and there is nothing I can do.*

I was feeling sad, angry and hopeless.

I lay in that stupid chair until about 6 a.m. I had barely slept and had completely lost my voice. I knew that I needed cough medicine with codeine. I used it years before and it had worked wonders. So I called my doctor's office and, hours later, I got a call from some doctor on-call who I didn't know. I explained my illness, growing rash and fear of taking the other medicine, and he said,

*"Sorry, I can't prescribe a narcotic over the phone. You can see your regular doctor on Tuesday since Monday is a holiday."*

I was annoyed. I told him I couldn't go another night without sleep; that I speak for a living and that I needed my voice.

*"Well, you can go to urgent care,"* he offered feebly.
*"Hope you feel better."*

We hung up and I was devastated. I was completely drained from all the energy it took to get dressed, and occupy Noam while Ron was sleeping. I ran to the bathroom and allowed the tears to flow. I saw Ron start to move but I didn't want to wake him. I thought:

*Will he ever get up?!*

I went back to the living room and sat close to Noam while the tears quietly streamed down my face. Noam noticed but didn't say a word. When Ron finally woke up and saw me, the tears flowed heavily. He held me as I tried to explain the sequence of events but I could barely speak. He was so sweet; he listened and actually empathized (not usually his strong point). Ron suggested we call our doctor-friend Ira. He couldn't prescribe me anything but referred us to a practice that is open on Sundays.

I called and spoke to an efficient nurse practitioner who asked a lot of detailed, intelligent questions. I told her that cough medicine with codeine had worked in the past, and she said,

*"That is exactly what we normally prescribe. Let me talk to the doctor for you."*

About 15 minutes later, she called me back with the green light. I had what I wanted – the good drugs without having to pay to see a doctor. Hallelujah!!!

Ron graciously picked up the cough medicine. I lay in bed for about 20 minutes after taking the syrup, and my cough subsided. I could feel relief as I started to doze off; I also had the sudden realization that my livelihood depends on my voice. Whether used for speaking or singing, my voice had always been the "gentle strength" that has allowed me to inspire freedom in others.

*Suddenly it dawned on me that I had been living my dream for quite some time!*

Even though I wanted to be earning more money, I loved my work and the impact I was having on peoples' lives.

The cough syrup was definitely helping although I can't function when taking it. Oh the joys of narcotics! But I had completely lost my voice. I could barely whisper, and I had a band rehearsal the next morning for a party I would be leading in 10 days. I prayed my voice would be restored by the next day but, by that evening, I realized that particular miracle would not be occurring. The band leader was very nice and understanding about the whole thing.

Okay, the next hurdle: I was expected to facilitate a morning session in Palm Springs for a Human Resources Association meeting in three days.

*Could I do it?*
*Could I perform?*

I felt obligated to make the event, and didn't want to cancel at the last minute. I emailed the meeting chairperson to let her know that I would do everything in my power to get there with a voice.

Although I was starting to heal, I still had a terrible cough. My mom convinced me to take antibiotics and my other dear doctor friend, Sharon, was kind enough to prescribe antibiotics for me. Thank God for her!

On Tuesday morning, the day I was heading to Palm Springs, my voice was barely more than a whisper but I managed to facilitate a good coaching session by phone. I decided to be gentle with myself and lay down for 30 minutes before heading out for the three-hour drive to Palm Springs.

When I woke up, I experienced a strange adrenalin rush; I had an inner knowing that everything was going to be all right. I walked around my house as I was getting dressed saying,

*I have this feeling everything is going to be all right. I am not sure why, but I feel a boost of energy and confidence and I am going to go with it. I am so appreciative of what we have. I know we will be okay. I will make it to Palm Springs, my voice will kick in.*

I felt short of breath and I could feel a flurry of activity in my stomach. It was such an odd sensation. I had my hot tea, medications, cough drops, and tissues all ready for my journey, and I was literally about to leave when my phone rang. The caller ID showed "Suntrust Mortgage" – the company that serviced our mortgage, the one I had been battling for a solid year to approve our loan modification. The last time I had spoken to someone there, he had turned us down flat. He had been very rude and the call abruptly ended with me in tears. We had resubmitted our request through our attorney and had been waiting for months. Hmm, Suntrust Mortgage –

*Am I up to this call?*
*Why do these calls come directly to me and not to Ron?*
*Do I want to answer the phone??*

I decided to answer it, and a woman named Amy told me our loan modification had been APPROVED!!

*Approved?? Could it really be so?*

My heart was pounding and my thoughts were racing. I tried to calm down enough to ask the right questions. I asked:

*"What is your contact information, Amy? I don't believe we have spoken before. What are the loan terms? When do we need to sign the paperwork and send it in with a certified check?"*

I went through all the pertinent details I could think of and hung up the phone. I had been waiting for that call for more than a year! I realized that our attorney knew someone at the bank, which is the only reason the deal had gone through. I sat there in shock and disbelief.

*Did that really just happen??*

What really amazed me was that my body and soul knew something was up. I now understood as I realized moments before that call, I had a kind of weird, nervous inner-knowing. Wow! Now the big questions that had been on hold for months would have to be answered:

*Can we afford the loan terms?*
*Should we declare bankruptcy?*

And the big one:

*Do we move to Israel?*

I immediately called Ron and shared the news.
"*Shit,*" he declared.

"*Why 'shit'? Aren't you happy even for a moment that it went through?*"

Right off, he started philosophizing as if all the drama was now over.

"*This chapter is now behind us,*" he said.
"*Even though applying for the modification was very stressful and cost us a lot, it was worth it.*"

And then, he hit me with:

"*I guess I'll call the attorney and the realtor to sell the house so we can move to Israel.*"
"*What?!*" I asked. "*Please don't call the realtor.*"

He just laughed and said,

"*Don't worry. I won't call the realtor...yet.*"

After we hung up, my immediate thoughts were,

*Can't we somehow make the terms of the loan work?*
*Can't we stay in America or do we have to move to Israel?*

How interesting that Ron's first thoughts were to call the realtor so we could start the process of moving to Israel. I had the opposite feeling that I wanted to stay here in the U.S. It had taken us so long to get those new terms approved.

I left for Palm Springs thinking and praying I would be able to identify and read the signs that could help me determine our next steps. I listened to every song on the radio as if it held a secret message for me to decode. I thought,

> *Does this song mean we should move to Israel?*
> *Does that song mean I would be happy if we move to Israel?*

After awhile, I gave up and let my mind drift since the answers weren't coming and I needed to focus on having a voice the next morning.

After arriving in Palm Springs, I checked into my hotel and walked across the street to find a restaurant. That little walk required a great deal of effort but I was grateful to have had the energy to walk at all. I found a nice French bistro in a strip mall (how strange!), and enjoyed a good dinner despite my coughing attacks. Once back at the hotel, I took my cough medicine with codeine and prayed for the best in the morning.

I woke up coughing and with every cough I felt like I was stabbing my vocal chords and that I wouldn't be able to speak or sing again. I took a shower to let the steam fill my lungs. I started to loosen up and was ready to face the day.

Amazingly my body cooperated with me. My voice was soft and crackly but I made it through. Ironically, I was speaking on the topic of "self-resilience" as the key to working through change. I had certainly been resilient in making it to that speaking engagement, and I spoke from my heart. I could feel the participants opening up and warming up. They freely participated, and I saw them resonating with me and my topic. I was vulnerable and authentic with them. I knew the morning had been a great success and that I had motivated people in a meaningful way. That is why I love my work — I get to touch and impact people's lives on a deeply personal level.

I was so grateful that I had made it through and that my voice had held out. I actually think that my having a weak voice may have endeared me to the participants, making them feel even closer to me. Yet another example of how being vulnerable and transparent can be a strength that brings people together versus a weakness. I was relieved that I could head home and maybe even catch a nap before having to pick up the kids. I still had major life decisions to make but for the time being, I was just grateful to be alive.

## Lessons Learned

Our bodies send us powerful information if we listen carefully. Our challenge is that our brain sometimes operates in opposition to our body. It lies and tells us we need to keep going, continue to push forward, no matter what. We become slaves to our brains.

My body spoke loud and clear to me during this experience. It yelled "slow down." "You are not superwoman!"

This experience was highly enlightening as I recognized that I had been living my so called dream for quite a while. I acknowledged my blessings especially my gentle strength – my voice. I realized that I need to nurture my voice so that I can continue to work and thrive. My voice is my livelihood.

I also experienced a deep inner knowing that I along with my family would be all right. My Performer kicks in when I face adversity.

## Deepen Your Learning

1. **What are you grateful for in your life?**

   _____
   _____
   _____
   _____

2. **What are you taking for granted in your life? Where is there room to show appreciation and gratitude?**

   _____
   _____
   _____
   _____

3. How self-resilient are you currently? Describe a situation where you thrived despite the challenges you faced? What actions did you take? Who were you being that allowed you to be successful?

   _____
   _____
   _____
   _____

4. Describe a time you had an inner knowing and you listened to the message. What was the experience like? What was the result?

   _____
   _____
   _____
   _____

# 20
## A New Chapter Begins – the Best is Yet to Come

Much has shifted in my life since I began writing this book:

- Ron landed a new job and was earning commission. He got laid off after two years and was looking for work again. He recently started selling roofing services and is really enjoying the work. He is starting to make money again too – yay!
- Our home-loan modification went through and we are close to finishing a debt-consolidation process to rebuild our credit. I recently got approved for a car lease and two credit cards – yippee!!
- My business has picked up considerably and I am working like a crazy person (of course, as a consultant, one never knows how long it will last). I am happy to share this has been my most successful year to date!
- I have adjusted to my gluten-free lifestyle and am at peace with my new eating regimen. I am still getting rashes and trying to figure out either how to prevent them and/or to treat them more effectively.
- Talia was accepted into a Jewish high school and was able to attend due to an incredible scholarship coupled with Ron's parents' amazing generosity.

I am truly grateful that these key foundational elements have taken shape.

After our loan modification had come through, it became very clear to me that I was not ready to uproot my family and move to Israel. I shared my decision with Ron and needless to say, he was pretty upset about the fact that we won't be moving now. I told him that I don't want to create more upheaval now that the pieces are coming together, and that I don't feel we can move to Israel just because he wants to be close to family and thinks it would be good for the kids. He won't suddenly become happier or more fulfilled just by living closer to his family; he has inner work to do to be clearer about who he is and what he wants. I am not ready to risk such a large move without his having clarity on these issues. He concurred with my perspective although it saddens him and he agreed to continue to seek counseling.

It's funny how the story continues to unfold: my Perfectionist began writing this book with the intention of having a happy ending but once into the writing process, my life took an unexpected turn that was — and continues to be — messy and difficult. But then my Performer kicked in and I became extremely creative. My Professional served me by giving me the grace to hold my head high and find the right things to say. I mustn't forget that it was my Perfectionist that drove me to take action in the first place. The experience forced me to throw my fears out the window and just go for it. I turned on the music full blast in my professional world by singing during training and speaking engagements and my singing continues to bring me tremendous joy and encouragement.

So, the lessons are finally becoming clearer. Of course, I would have appreciated learning them a little sooner and with a lot less pain. I continue to embrace my "gentle strength" and allow my Performer to take the lead as much as possible. I now know that I am most successful and fulfilled when I am grounded in my authenticity. I resonate with people the most when I show them my heart and let them see me for me – flaws and all.

I continue to marvel at the power of vulnerability and how this works in opposition to perfectionism. Most people consider vulnerability to be a weakness. This is obvious even by looking at simple definitions of vulnerability –

1) "capable of or susceptible to being wounded or hurt, as by a weapon: **Example**: *a vulnerable part of the body.*"

2) "open to moral attack, criticism, temptation, etc.: **Example**: *He is vulnerable to bribery.*"

There are great risks when we are vulnerable including fear of being rejected and the potential for opening up old wounds. Being vulnerable can trigger us to subconsciously recall past traumas. The brain feels as if that trauma is happening now.

So why am I encouraging you to be vulnerable with so much at stake? There are actually many **rewards** when we are vulnerable including:

1) Increased self-awareness which builds connection within ourselves and others.

2) Being in alignment and living an integrated life. We experience tremendous joy and fulfillment when we are living "on purpose."

3) Being authentic and real. This provides opportunities to ask for what we want so we can pursue our dreams. This leads to living a juicier life.

Being vulnerable can actually be a strength and a key to leading an authentic, fulfilling life. Perfectionism on the other hand demands that we hide key aspects of ourselves due to a variety of reasons including fear, shame, insecurity, etc. Perfectionism is an attempt to control who we are so we won't experience failure or pain. It is impossible to be vulnerable and a perfectionist at the same time. They are in contradiction to one another.

I realize that I continue to battle between the old tapes of perfectionism and the deeper knowing that I experience my greatest joys and triumphs when I let go, surrender, and allow myself to vulnerable. Listening to that deeper voice requires courageousness and trust. The more I build the muscle of listening to that inner knowing, the easier it is for me to shift the irrational beliefs of my perfectionism.

Will I have the strength to continue to follow my authentic path? I certainly plan to, and I am excited to see where it leads.

How does this all apply to you the reader?

I hope you have found my story to be inspiring. My prayer and wish for you is that you find and honor your inner voice. May you (and I) connect to your authentic values, passions, and dreams so that you can live a more integrated life. In other words, once you know what is important to you, how can you incorporate this into every aspect of your life? Enough with compartmentalizing and wearing a mask! How can you authentically shine in all areas of life?

I also trust that you realize that life truly is a journey with ups and downs, twists, and turns. Perfection does not exist. We are better served being vulnerable, striving for excellence and doing our best. When we do this we are able to turn our messes into our messages instead of shoving them into an overflowing drawer we pray no one will ever open.

Trust that things happen for a reason and that you have the strength to break through your fears and truly flourish. Stop focusing on what you cannot control and instead pay attention to where you can be in charge and what you can influence. One of the few things we can control is our attitude. Of course this is not such an easy thing to do AND it is important to remember that by changing our perspective, we will alter our thoughts, emotions, and therefore our actions.

May you embrace all of who you are so that you can thrive in every aspect of your life. So be it...

## Lessons Learned

There are no coincidences in life. I continue to be presented with some tough circumstances. I was tasked with discovering the learning from these painful experiences. My fear pushed me into action and I was able to more fully embrace my Performer and just GO FOR IT! I realized this was my best chance at being successful. There was no room for paralysis.

I am amazed how all the pieces continue to come together and that I am thriving personally and professionally. These events over the last three years have changed my perspective and have helped me find the strength and courage to live from my heart and let my Performer take the lead more frequently.

## Deepen Your Learning

1. **What do you absolutely trust about yourself?**

   _____
   _____
   _____
   _____
   _____

2. **Reflect on how perfectionism and vulnerability operate in your world. Which voice do you tend to follow and why?**

   _____
   _____
   _____
   _____
   _____

3. Commit to one action you can accomplish in the next two weeks to propel you forward personally and/or professionally. Write down the action and how you will hold yourself accountable.

_____
_____
_____
_____
_____

# In Gratitude

I feel appreciation and gratitude to so many people that supported me in creating this meaningful project.

Thanks to my friends and family for consenting to share the stories and adventures we have experienced together.

Thanks to my friends and supporters including Jean, Lori, Daphne, Sharon, Kim, Carol, Kathie, John, Robyn, and Judith who were involved with reading my book, providing feedback and, have spent much time empathizing with me as I wrote my story.

Thanks to Mary for your ongoing support and incredible generosity.

Thanks to one of my dearest friends Maria for continually and patiently sharing her wisdom, encouraging me to pursue my dreams, and who provided input on the book title and cover.

My thank you list would not be complete without acknowledging my friend Dawn. Without her, where would I be? I never would have pursued physical therapy which ultimately led to my reconnecting with performing.

A special thanks to my amazing support team including my editors Kim Rahilly and Kevin Ramirez, my publishing guru Juliet Clark, my public relations specialist Pavarti K Tyler, and my graphic artists Dev Karna, and Kimberly Martin.

I also want to acknowledge myself for my commitment to this project although it took more time to complete than my Perfectionist desired. I want to thank my Performer for giving me the strength to stand strong in my vulnerability. I am grateful for my intuition – my gentle strength that continues to remind me to courageously live from my heart.

## About the Author

Rachel Karu's quest for an authentic, inspirational life led her to found RAE Development - a professional and personal development practice. An experienced coach, speaker, trainer, and singer with over 19 years' experience, she energizes her clients and creates an affirming environment for personal and professional transformation. Prior to launching RAE Development, Rachel served as Human Resources Manager at EMI Music Distribution and the Manager of Organization Development and Training at Easton Sports, Inc.

Rachel earned a Master of Science in Counseling for Business, Industry and Government and a Bachelor of Science in Business with a specialization in Human Resources. She achieved her Coaching Credential through the International Coaching Federation. Rachel is certified/qualified in a variety of assessment tools including the Myers Briggs Type Indicator. Clients include: Raytheon, United States Navy, U.S. Marine Corps, Nestle, Citibank, Allergan, Tenet Healthcare, Philips, Braille Institute, Mattel, Viacom, and Disney/ABC Media. Rachel is happily married to an amazing soul mate and is the proud mom of two incredible kids!

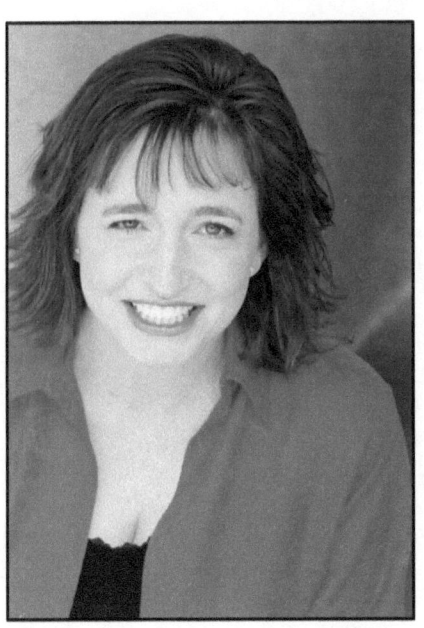

www.ingramcontent.com/pod-product-compliance
Lightning Source LLC
Chambersburg PA
CBHW030233170426
43201CB00006B/205